MEN OVER 50 GET HEALTHY

STEADFAST STRATEGIES FOR LONGEVITY AND AGING WELL

JACKSON MCNEIL

CONTENTS

INTRODUCTION

Are you truly as healthy as you believe? The startling revelations about your well-being that accompany aging might leave you pondering. A significant number of us live under the false comfort of perceived wellness – a mirage that fades as age etches its indelible lines. Suddenly, an everyday activity strains your muscles, or a regular visit to the physician ends with advice for a radical dietary transformation to fend off cardiac issues. While aging can indeed be daunting, it doesn't have to cloud your existence if you seize the current moment to take charge of your health and steer toward a healthier lifestyle.

In the whirlwind of modern society, a large number of men in their middle ages unknowingly fall into the grip of unhealthy aging. They are lured by the unbridled appeal of instant solutions that often turn out to be temporary Band-Aids, cunningly designed to keep them coming back. Wrestling with the physical impacts of aging, they yearn for a life-altering approach but are left in the shadows, uncertain of which direction to take.

This book offers itself as your thorough guide to not merely surviving the storm of middle age but thriving within its trials. By embracing the methods proposed within this book, you stand to gain an array of advantages: an extended lifespan, rejuvenated energy, improved cognitive abilities and memory, a lower risk of chronic diseases – the benefits seem endless. However, the key takeaway here is this: investing in a healthy lifestyle can deliver remarkable rewards, enriching your life quality as you traverse the path of aging.

Within these pages, you'll discover answers to pressing concerns such as, "How can I boost my overall wellness?" and "What changes can I bring to my diet to bolster my health?" and "How can I integrate regular physical activity into my daily routine?" and many more. Yet, the true purpose of this manuscript goes beyond delivering mere advice and strategies. Its core objective is to aid you in designing a viable plan aimed at achieving optimal health and, in the process, a deep sense of joy and satisfaction.

As a previous educator of physics and chemistry who has experienced a spectrum of unhealthy habits, both self-inflicted and inherited, I can relate to the health challenges men encounter. Like a reassembled *Six Million Dollar Man*, I've been reconstructed from scratch. But I've chosen not to let those health challenges dictate how I lead my life. Instead, I've resolved, within my means, to pursue health and longevity.

This book pinpoints the prevalent and extensively studied health problems that most men in their middle ages (50+) face. It provides authentic strategies and inspiration to fight the effects of aging and to mitigate the risks of declining health. It's not a broad dissertation on men's health filled with unspecific pearls of wisdom and generic directives encouraging the continuation of behaviors leading to your current state of health. The old saying, "Dance with the one that brought you," doesn't apply here. It's time to find a new dance partner.

A considerable number of middle-aged men lead an unhealthy existence. Doubtful? Just look around. Nearly 40% of men aged 51+ are overweight or obese. If you underestimate your significance, not just for your own sake, but for your family, spouse, partner, children – to name a few – then you need to realize, YOU MATTER! You influence the world in innumerable, even if unnoticeable, ways. Your interactions with clients, store attendants, your children – the list goes on – shape the way people perceive and react to the world. Your worth is indisputable. You deserve to dedicate time to self-care and your health. Attaining and maintaining good health doesn't have to be expensive. All it requires is a deliberate decision to prioritize it.

In a world that can be negligent about health, we've come to accept poor conditions as inevitable consequences of getting older. But it doesn't have to be that way. My experience of overcoming my own health issues has empowered me with the knowledge and the tools that I believe can make a difference in your life. This book, therefore, serves as a practical manual for all middle-aged men seeking to turn the tables on their health.

This book doesn't deliver arbitrary advice or impossible demands. Instead, it provides a comprehensive exploration of the health problems middle-aged men face. It offers strategies for dealing with them head-on, making lifestyle changes, and paving the way to optimal health. It isn't a theoretical discourse; it is a real, practical guide for health, designed from personal experiences and meticulous research.

Most importantly, it aims to create a mindset shift. Rather

than dreading the health problems that may come with age, it guides you on how to embrace the journey and turn it into a celebration of life. It drives home the point that aging need not be a countdown to illness, but rather can be an excellent opportunity to improve and enjoy life more fully.

The investment you make in your health today is the foundation for a healthier, happier tomorrow. Whether it's about diet, exercise, or attitude, the changes you make today can have profound effects on your health and overall quality of life. So, I encourage you to take the first step toward a healthier lifestyle. Let this book guide you along the path of self-improvement, self-care, and healthier aging.

Let's commence this transformative journey to health with the first chapter, "Your Health, Your Party." It's time to dance to a new tune, one that celebrates life and wellness. Embrace the chance to reinvent yourself and your health because it is, after all, your party. Your health is a treasure, and you are worth every effort to preserve and enhance it.

The companion, *"Men Over 50 Get Healthy Workbook"* is designed to serve as a dedicated space for you to meticulously record your thoughts, reflections, and any insightful data gathered during your health transformation journey. Whether used in tandem with the book or as an independent resource, it is a purposeful tool to foster your introspection and enhance your progress. This product is conceived to inspire and facilitate your dedication toward achieving holistic health.

You can receive my newsletter and blog at jacksonmcneil.com

NAVIGATING THE PASSAGE TO DYNAMIC AGING – YOUR HEALTH – YOUR PARTY

"Age is an issue of mind over matter. If you don't mind, it doesn't matter."
– Mark Twain

I n this never-ending dance of life, Twain's timeless wisdom echoes with renewed understanding. Amid the turmoil that life can often present, I sometimes disregard my own well-being until a slap of fate delivers me a vivid reality check. I recall feeling indestructible, sprinting through life with unbridled passion. Growing up for me was the ultimate prize, an opportunity to carve out my calling and captain my own ship. Now, I crave the simplicity of those long-gone, carefree, and uncomplicated days. Regrettably, they vanished faster than a shadow on a cloudy day. Time has seasoned me, and with it surfaces the realization that my trusty body can no longer withstand my youthful shenanigans. Although I can't turn back the clock, I can wholeheartedly embrace the years to come, discovering strength and pleasure in the unfolding adventure.

Aging is inescapable, etching itself on my face, pilfering my hair's boyish hue (what's left of it), and inconveniencing my body with demands that I am, at times, unable to answer. However, with a committed mindset and a determination, I can sail through aging with style and strength.

As I look back, I long for the body I once had, secretly suspecting it has been swapped with this creaky, groaning vessel gazing back at me in the mirror every morning. But remember, growing older is a privilege denied to many. So, as I throw my doubts away and tackle this new chapter head-on, I will claim my place in the dazzling pantheon of silver-maned foxes and golden gods. I steady myself and sometimes stumble into this uncharted territory, gazing in the face of adversity, relishing in my triumphs, and proving that life after 50 is dynamic, full of surprises, and never boring. With steadfast resolve and shrewd strategies, I find that life's most exceptional moments are still waiting to unfold before me.

FACING THE MYSTERY OF AGING

Time's progression demands unbending determination; it can be a maze of consternation and doubt about our unknown future. But we are not alone. Research reveals (BMC Geriatrics, 2021) that untold numbers of men share our reservations. We have an obligation to push ahead, equipped with resolve to maintain our physical and mental competence, and to cultivate the relationships that help support us. We owe it not only to ourselves, but also to the people who love us and need us. The aging men of this world form the frontline in this struggle against time, confronting the oncoming waves that only age can present, often struggling with quiet discomfort. Recognizing the predictable march of time, it is time to adapt, rise, and meet its daily trials head-on.

DECIPHERING THE PUZZLE – CONFRONTING THE FEAR OF AGING

Beneath the surface, the fear of aging strikes deep into our essence. Our minds can sometimes create a complex picture of what our future looks like as we get older:

- *Fear of loss:* As time slips away, we're unsettled by the prospect of losing loved ones, abilities, and independence.
- *Fear of loneliness:* Time's passage may thin our ranks, leaving us isolated and craving for the fellowship of past days.
- *Fear of the unknown:* The road ahead is obscured in hazy uncertainty, and at times we get nervous before the unknowable future.
- *Negative social representation:* Society portrays aging as a descent into decay, provoking our fears and distorting our perceptions of the inevitable.
- *Fear of financial insecurity:* Retirement looms large, and the potential loss of income can cause anxiety for us and our families.
- *Fear of cognitive decline:* Time's effects do not spare the mind, and we have to confront the prospect of losing memories and wit.

- *Fear of losing one's identity:* As roles and responsibilities shift, we dread the erosion of the very core of who we are.

Understanding these fears and addressing them head-on can help us embrace the aging process with a more positive outlook. By actively challenging societal stereotypes and prioritizing our well-being, we can alleviate some of these concerns and better enjoy our golden years.

THE DOUBLE STANDARD OF AGING THEORY

I often wonder why we fear aging so intensely. Part of the answer lies in the "double standard of aging theory," which suggests that culture treats aging differently for men and women (Jones, 2020). Society's view of aging is complex and, at times, prejudicial. While some earn praise for maintaining a youthful and spirited appearance, others face stigma for exhibiting signs of age. This phenomenon, known as the "double standard of aging theory," impacts individuals across genders, races, and social classes.

You may have encountered this double standard on your passage to getting older. Age may have cost you career opportunities, or you may have felt overlooked in social situations due to society's narrow standards of beauty and youth. While men are often seen as becoming more distinguished and wiser with age (which create their own set of issues), women, on the other hand, are more likely to be judged by their appearance and considered less attractive (Jones, 2020). This disparity in how aging is perceived can fuel anxieties about growing older for both men and women.

Another issue is that times have really changed. Remember when families, with grandparents, parents, and kids, all lived close by or even under the same roof? Well, that's not the norm anymore. Nowadays, taking care of your aging parents might not be on your radar.

Chances are you and your partner/spouse are both working hard to keep up with the increasing cost of living in today's world. Finding the time and resources to care for your parents? That's no easy task. And let's not forget that you might be working well into your 70s just to stay relevant in your job.

As we get older, we've got a lot of stuff to deal with. Should our health be one of those problems? You can answer that for yourself.

Here's the silver lining: we can transform our perspective on aging and concentrate on the good things that come with experience and wisdom. By taking control of our health and embracing this trek in the wilderness, we can redefine what it means to age and make the most of our remaining years.

HEALTHY AGING VERSUS UNHEALTHY AGING – CHOOSE YOUR PATH WISELY

Recall those "Choose Your Own Adventure" books? You'd flip to different pages based on the decisions you made, hoping not to encounter a grisly fate. Life after 50 is somewhat similar, except the choices you make now determine whether you'll age like a fine wine or a bag of moldy cheese. As we explore the distinctions between healthy and unhealthy aging, the significance of making informed decisions about our lifestyle habits cannot be overlooked.

CHARACTERISTICS AND ADVANTAGES OF HEALTHY AGING

Physical Health: Envision yourself at 80, spending time playing with your grandkids, going on hikes, getting in 18 holes of golf with energy to spare, or even running a marathon. Sound too good to be true? It isn't if you prioritize your physical health (Smith et al., 2019). Healthy aging necessitates a few actions on your part: regular exercise, maintaining a healthy weight, and staying current with preventive healthcare. You'll be more energetic, have a robust immune system, and reduce the risk of developing chronic diseases like heart disease, diabetes, osteoporosis – you can fill in the blank for your affliction.

I come from a heritage of long-lived people – my mother, still kickin' into her 90s, and my dad's family into their 80s and 90s; so I'm cursed/blessed with a long life. I can't imagine being in my late 70s and not able to live the way I envision. Little to no energy, pain and joint issues, inflammation everywhere, all because I wasn't willing to take care of what I could when I could with my health.

Mental Well-Being: Healthy aging isn't solely about your body; it's also about your mind. Keeping your brain engaged through hobbies, puzzles, or acquiring new skills can help maintain cognitive function as you age (National Institute on Aging, n.d.). Mental well-being also involves managing stress, nurturing social connections, and getting sufficient sleep. Trust me, you'll not only want to attend parties instead of hitting the sack, but you'll also impress others with your sharpness well into your 60s, 70s, and 80s.

CHARACTERISTICS AND CONSEQUENCES OF UNHEALTHY AGING

Now, imagine the alternative: unhealthy aging. It's like watching your favorite movie star lose their charm, age poorly, and wonder, "What the hell happened?" Unhealthy aging can result from a lack of exercise, poor diet, smoking, excessive alcohol use, or neglecting preventive healthcare. (Smith et al., 2019) The consequences? Increased risk of chronic diseases, frailty, and cognitive decline (Smith et al., 2019). You might find yourself spending more time with your doctor than your friends, and nobody wants that.

The good news is that you have the power to choose how you age. It's never too late to make positive changes and reap the benefits. So, trade in the TV remote for a pair of sneakers and swap out the nightly wine, beer, or bourbon for a glass of water. Your future self will thank you. Take a look at what you've gained over the years and what it can mean for your future.

- *A Head and Heart Full of Wisdom and Knowledge*: you have a boundless reservoir of intellect and intuition, filled drop by drop with the passing of time. It is a priceless asset, full of life's lessons learned through hard times, failures, but always intended to give you the wisdom only age can produce.
- *Bonds of Steel*: As time marches on, we have refined our focus on relationships that truly enrich our lives. This evolution has created a life of profound, enduring connections with those we cherish most – our family and friends.

- *A Masterpiece of Self*: The path of aging gives us a true understanding of the uniqueness of our life. Its strengths, limitations, and self-awareness award us with unshakeable (at times) confidence and a clear sense of self.

MEDICINES AS A BAND-AID SOLUTION VERSUS FIXING THE PROBLEM

Take a Pill or Tackle the Issue?

In this fast-paced world, we crave instant gratification, seeking speedy solutions for just about everything. Sadly, this mindset has infiltrated our health, with many opting for prescription drugs as Band-Aid fixes instead of confronting the core issues. But, as we're about to discover, excessive reliance on medications can spawn a new set of predicaments.

Picture this: you're at a party, nursing a raging headache from the noise, work week, or the trials of raising teenagers – take your pick. You pop a painkiller, over-the-counter or prescription, and voilà, problem solved! Right? In this land of liberty, we like shortcuts, especially when it comes to health. We often depend on our friends Jack or Tito to make our woes vanish – albeit temporarily.

As a nation, we're the world's biggest consumers of prescription painkillers. Working Partners reveals that the United States, boasting a mere 4.4% of the global population, swallows a staggering 80% of the planet's opioid supply and 99% of its hydrocodone. But our love affair doesn't end there; we're also infatuated with antibiotics, antidepressants, and an array of other meds.

The issue? These quick fixes often target symptoms, neglecting the underlying problems. While we might experience short-term relief, we're not genuinely addressing the root causes of our health concerns. Over-reliance on medications, as the saying goes, too much of a good thing can turn bad if not properly managed. Such dependence can bring on adverse drug reactions, addiction, and even more health complications (Merck Manual, 2020). The Merck Manual notes that adults in their 50s are particularly susceptible to the detrimental effects of excessive medication use, as they often juggle multiple drugs for various health conditions (Merck Manual, 2020).

So, we stand at a crossroads, faced with a choice: transient comfort or lasting solutions. By tackling the root causes of our ailments, we can break free from the restraints of medication dependence and lay the foundation for a more vibrant, practical existence.

I'm not going to dwell on the doom and gloom because growing older comes with abundant perks. One strategy for achieving better health is appreciating and celebrating the positives of aging. Embrace the wisdom, experience, and connections that come with the passing years, and let them guide you toward a healthier, more fulfilling life.

THE IMPORTANCE OF ADDRESSING ROOT CAUSES OF HEALTH ISSUES

Rather than leaning on medications to conceal our health problems, we can concentrate on tackling the root causes. Hanging onto a more holistic approach to our well-being includes eating as healthy as we're able, regular exercise, stress management, and laughing at yourself from time to time.

Allow me to illustrate with a few examples. If you're dealing with high blood pressure, prescription medication may offer temporary relief. I'm not suggesting you abandon your doctor-prescribed medication; instead, have a frank conversation with your physician about alternative solutions for your specific health concern. A more workable strategy would involve modifying your diet, increasing physical activity, and managing stress levels.

Similarly, if you're feeling down, an antidepressant may provide some relief, but it won't resolve the underlying causes of your depression. For people with clinical depression, it is imperative that they should always consult their doctor. There are health strategies that are a great adjunct and tactic to their anti-depressant and may enable them to taper down on dosage. However, pursuing therapy, nurturing social connections, and exploring personal interests are also effective long-term strategies.

So, let's be rational and thoughtful about discarding quick fixes, by rolling up our sleeves, and confronting our health issues directly. We're not merely aiming for a longer life – we're pursuing a happier, healthier one too.

YOUR WELLNESS WORKBOOK – ENGAGING TASKS FOR A HEALTHIER YOU

Gentlemen, it's time to get down to business and face the challenge. Though building a deck, or cleaning out the garage, or even, God forbid, plumbing repairs may seem more manageable, I'm talking about the core of the matter – our health. So, grab a pen, find the accompanying workbook/journal to this book, and let's begin. I'll guide you through essential steps to help you reflect on your personal health journey, fears, and defining moments. The time for change is now, and this is where it all begins.

Starting your health holiday, you may sneer at the thought of a workbook or journal. "Seriously? I'm not a teenager jotting down feelings about the latest boy band." But bear with me. Journaling isn't solely about emotional expression – it's about self-discovery, reflection, and goal setting. It has proven to be a potent instrument for tracking progress and maintaining accountability. Writing out your ideas and what is going on in your head helps clarify your thought process and will bring out your focus. It will legitimize your feelings and thinking, your self-reflections, and attitudes about change. You must be convinced in your own head and heart, not only of the impor-tance of your health, but what it means to those who care about you.

Set aside a few minutes each day to write in your journal. Record your health goals, progress, setbacks, and victories. Be brutally honest with yourself. This journal is exclusively for you, so there's no need to sugarcoat anything. As you continue on your health odyssey, you'll discover that revisiting your entries can offer invaluable insights and motivation to propel you forward. The most important question you must answer is why. What is your why? For success to happen, your motivation is paramount to seeing the change you want and need, resolving the "why" is the beginning.

As a former Chemistry and Physics teacher, I would have to remind my students that "they" are in charge of their brain. Their brain doesn't decide their choices, "they" do. So, take control and do it.

Imagine standing at the edge of a cliff, watching a cascade of water flowing into a serene, crystal-clear pool below. You can feel the warmth of the sun, your lungs filled with the invigorating scent of the surrounding forest as the mist from the waterfall gently cools your face. At the bottom of the cliff is a world of newfound energy, mental clarity, and physical well-being. This is the world that making your health a priority can open for you.

But as you stand there, contemplating whether to take the plunge, you hesitate. You're busy and making such a big change seems daunting. So, you decide to stay where you are, clinging to the comfort of your current habits.

As time goes on, you start to feel the ground beneath you crumble. The lively colors around you begin to fade, and the air becomes still. You can no longer feel the refreshing mist from the waterfall, and the pool below looks further and further away.

By choosing not to engage in exercise and healthy living, you are surrendering to a world of missed opportunities. It's not just about the immediate loss of energy, focus, and well-being, but also about the long-term consequences of that decision. You might find yourself troubled by chronic health issues, mental fatigue, and decreased productivity. The comfort of inaction, once so appealing, now feels like a weight that you can't shake off.

It becomes evident that the price of inaction is much higher than the effort required to take the plunge. Don't let the fear of change hold you back from experiencing the full, vibrant life that exercise and healthy living can bring. It's not just a missed opportunity; it's a step away from the person you could become.

KEY TAKEAWAYS

1. Overcome fears and challenges of aging by understanding their roots.
2. Choose healthy lifestyle habits for a better aging experience.
3. Avoid over-reliance on medicines and address health issues at their core.
4. Reflect on personal fears and defining moments to start a health journey.
5. Empower yourself by taking charge of your health, no matter your age.

FINAL THOUGHTS

Getting old can be intimidating, but it doesn't have to be. We've explored the various fears and challenges that come with aging, and how to overcome them. We've also looked at the benefits of healthy aging and the potential consequences of unhealthy aging. And we've learned about the dangers of over-reliance on medicines and the importance of addressing root causes of health issues. The key takeaway is it's never too late to take charge of your health and well-being. Like my buddy Wayne says, "If I knew I was gonna live this long, I would've taken better care of myself." Our bodies are incredibly resilient and able to withstand years of abuse, but there comes a time when the jig is up, and we know inside it's time to make this happen.

So, with conscious choices and a commitment to a healthy life-style, you can set yourself up for a long, healthy, and happy life.

Now that you understand how important healthy aging is, let's explore the concept of longevity and how you can prepare for it. In the next chapter, we'll discuss the science of longevity and the secrets of those who live to a healthy ripe old age. Get ready to be inspired and motivated to make the most of the rest of your life.

2

LONGEVITY – MYTH OR REALITY

You're reclining on your sofa, a bowl of popcorn within arm's reach, enthusiastically consuming the latest season of your favorite show. You had intended on going for a walk or hitting the gym, but the magnetic pull of the television screen was simply irresistible. "Ah, what's one more laid-back day, eh?"

But here's the crux: every decision we make, monumental or minute, initiates a domino effect, shaping our future. It's these seemingly insignificant choices that have guided you to your current position. And it's by making more judicious choices that we can form the future we long for.

Again, "If only I knew I'd live this long, I would've taken better care of myself." It's a widely shared sentiment, but it's never too late to put your well-being first. In this chapter, we'll probe the correlation between happiness and health and how more shrewd choices can lead to a more robust, contented you.

THE UNHAPPY–UNHEALTHY CONNECTION

Were you aware that unhappiness can be detrimental? Unhappy people are susceptible to a surplus of physical and mental health issues (Smith et al., 2022). It's a vicious cycle: when you're feeling low, you're likely to make unhealthy choices, which, in turn, exacerbates your unhappiness.

So, how do your everyday decisions influence your overall happiness and health? In essence, they're everything. The choices you make, such as selecting a donut or a banana for breakfast or opting for the stairs over the elevator, profoundly affect your well-being. When you consistently make decisions that promote a healthy lifestyle, you're more likely to experience happiness and improved health.

The bright side is that it's never too late to start making better choices. By identifying the decisions that hinder you and replacing them with healthier options, you can chart a new course toward happiness and well-being. It all commences with acknowledging the patterns in your life that perpetuate unhappiness and then taking concrete steps to alter them. Of course, if it were that easy everyone would do it, right?

ROOT CAUSE ANALYSIS – UNEARTHING THE SOURCE OF UNHEALTHINESS

To boost your health and happiness, it's imperative to determine the root cause of your present circumstances. Root Cause Analysis (RCA) is a potent problem-solving method extensively employed in the business realm to discern the underlying causes of an issue (ASQ, n.d.). By applying RCA to your personal life, you can pinpoint the specific decisions and behaviors that contribute to your unhappiness and unhealthiness.

Before you read through this list, remember: the beginning stages of change can be a bit tedious and sometimes a pain-in-the-ass to get into. If you can struggle with and move through this first part, the enormity of change with not only your mindset and attitude, but also how quickly your body will respond to deliberate actions to get it repaired, will be worth every moment. Stick with it!

Here's a five-step process to execute an RCA:

1. *Define the problem*: Clearly express the issue at hand, such as unhappiness or unhealthiness. Be specific and avoid vague statements.
2. *Collect data*: Accumulate information about the problem, i.e., your daily habits, emotions, and thoughts that may be contributing to your current state.
3. *Identify possible causal factors*: Analyze the data and ascertain which factors could be causing your unhappiness and unhealthiness. These could include an unhealthy diet, insufficient exercise, or negative thought patterns.
4. *Identify the root cause(s)*: Delve deeper into the causal factors and determine the underlying cause(s) of the problem. This might involve revealing emotional triggers, past experiences, or deeply ingrained beliefs that affect your decisions and behaviors.
5. *Develop and implement a plan for change*: Once you've identified the root cause(s), devise a plan to tackle

them and enhance your overall well-being. This could involve setting goals, establishing new habits, or seeking professional help if necessary. Most importantly, commit to implementing the required changes and tracking your progress along the way.

Struggling to grasp the concept? Let's apply the five-step RCA to a common health and happiness issue: weight gain.

1. *Define the problem:* Over the past few years, you've gained weight, and it's impacting your happiness and overall well-being.
2. *Collect data:* You document your daily habits, such as your eating patterns, exercise regimen (or lack thereof), and emotional state.
3. *Identify possible causal factors:* Upon examining the data, you realize that your weight gain could be attributed to excessive snacking, a sedentary lifestyle, and emotional eating in response to stress.
4. Identify the root cause(s): With further introspection, you uncover that the root cause of your emotional eating and weight gain is your high-stress job, which has led to unhealthy coping mechanisms.
5. *Develop and implement a plan for change*: Armed with this newfound insight, you create a plan to address the root cause. This might include adopting healthier ways to manage stress, such as practicing mindfulness or seeking therapy, as well as adjusting your diet and exercise routine.

By utilizing RCA to identify the source of your unhealthiness, you can empower yourself to make informed decisions that will ultimately result in a happier, healthier you. The key is to be honest with yourself, be willing to confront the root causes of your unhappiness and commit to making the necessary changes.

Always bear in mind, you possess the power to sculpt your future, one decision at a time.

EXCUSES AND STAGNATION – CONQUERING MENTAL OBSTACLES

The mind is a formidable instrument. It can propel you toward success or be the very force impeding you. If you've ever found yourself trapped in a stalemate or incapable of making the changes you know are essential, it's likely that your mindset is playing a pivotal role. The encouraging news is that once you recognize the influence your thoughts have on your actions, you can take measures to alter them and ultimately enhance your life.

FREQUENT EXCUSES AND REBUTTALS AGAINST THEM

We all concoct excuses from time to time, but some are more prevalent than others. Here are some of the most recurrent excuses regarding health and happiness, accompanied by rebuttals against them:

- *"I don't have time to exercise."* In truth, you allocate time for the things that matter to you. If you can find time to indulge in your favorite TV series, you can likely spare 20-30 minutes a day for physical activity.

- *"I'm too exhausted to work out."* While it might be true that you're fatigued, studies indicate that exercise can elevate your energy levels (Harvard Health Publishing, 2021). Moreover, consistent physical activity can help you sleep better at night, resulting in less tiredness in the long run.
- *"I can't afford a gym membership."* Gym memberships can be expensive, but they aren't a necessity to get fit. There are innumerable free or low-cost resources available, such as online workout videos, local parks, and community centers.
- *"I don't know how to eat healthily."* With an abundance of information accessible online and in books, it's easier than ever to educate yourself on proper nutrition. Additionally, there are numerous simple, healthy recipes you can attempt that don't necessitate a culinary degree.

Now that we've debunked some common excuses, let's delve into strategies to help you surmount them and advance:

- *Reframe your thoughts:* Instead of concentrating on the barriers that hinder you, focus on the advantages of making healthier choices. For instance, rather than thinking, "I'm too tired to exercise," consider, "Exercising will give me more energy and improve my sleep quality."
- *Break goals into manageable steps:* Large objectives can be daunting, which is why breaking them down into

smaller, more attainable steps is crucial. If your goal is to lose 20 pounds, initiate by aiming to lose one pound per week.

- *Discover your motivation:* Identify what genuinely inspires you to make healthier choices. Is it the aspiration to live longer, feel better, or set a positive example for your children? Keep your motivation at the forefront of your mind as you strive toward your goals.

- *Be accountable:* Share your objectives with a supportive friend or family member, join a group with similar goals, or use an app to monitor your progress. Accountability can be a potent motivator in overcoming excuses and staying on course. Personally, I have given my wife permission to call me out when I make poor food choices. Usually, it's a look or a raised eyebrow, a bit irritating in the beginning, but very effective. Her health changes have inspired me to be much more conscious of my decisions about a healthy lifestyle.

ACTIVITIES TO FOSTER CHANGE

Armed with knowledge of Root Cause Analysis (RCA), it's time to apply it. Consider an aspect of your life where you'd like to see improvements and follow the five-step RCA process to pinpoint the root cause(s) and develop a plan for change (ASQ, n.d.).

After completing your RCA, identify two actionable steps to start addressing the root cause(s). These steps should be specific, measurable, and attainable. For instance, if your RCA revealed that stress is the primary cause of your unhealthy habits, two actionable steps might be to practice mindfulness meditation for ten minutes daily and schedule regular breaks throughout your workday.

Open up your workbook/journal and write down your three most common excuses for not making healthier choices. Then, employing the strategies discussed earlier, plan counterarguments for each excuse. Once you've accomplished this, ceremoniously burn the paper (safely and preferably outdoors) as a symbolic gesture of releasing these excuses and committing to change.

KEY TAKEAWAYS

1. Our past decisions shape our current health and happiness, but we have the power to make positive changes going forward.
2. Unhappiness and unhealthiness are interconnected and addressing one can lead to improvements in the other.
3. Root Cause Analysis (RCA) is a versatile tool that can help pinpoint the underlying issues in various aspects of our lives.
4. Recognizing and overcoming self-imposed limitations and excuses is crucial for personal growth and improvement.
5. Small, actionable steps can lead to significant, lasting changes in our health, happiness, and overall well-being.

FINAL THOUGHTS

As you conclude this chapter and advance, remember that you possess the power to transform your life. It's not about executing grand, sweeping changes overnight – it's about taking small, manageable steps every day that will steadily guide you towards a healthier, happier existence.

Embrace the insights and strategies shared in this chapter, and above all, believe in your ability to effect meaningful change. You are stronger, more resilient, and more capable than you may realize. As you begin to address the root causes of your unhappiness and unhealthiness, you'll uncover the power within you to surmount obstacles, liberate yourself from self-imposed constraints, and flourish.

Remember, your decisions today possess the power to mold your future. By modifying the small choices, you make each day, you can lay the foundation for the healthier, happier life you merit. So, forge ahead with determination, bravery, and optimism. Your drive towards a brighter, healthier future commences now.

In the following chapter, we'll delve into the fascinating realm of brain science to reveal tactics for making better choices that will not only enhance your health and happiness but also help you achieve greater success in every facet of your life.

3

YOUR WILL OVER THE PHYSICAL – THE POWER OF MIND OVER MATTER

When we say, "Mind Over Matter," we're talking about the astounding ability of our thoughts, attitude, and perception to influence our physical experiences and health. The idea isn't some magical mumbo-jumbo; it's rooted in the world of science, specifically within the realm of psychology and neuroscience. But how does it work?

In this chapter, I'm going to dive deep into the mental side of things. I'll explore how to stay mentally sharp, unlock motivation, and harness the power of a growth mindset to keep you pushing forward on your journey to better health.

The foundation of this philosophy rests on the premise that our mental state, our thoughts, emotions, and attitudes, can impact our physical state. For instance, ever noticed how stress can give you a headache, or how excitement can make your heart race? That's mind over matter at work. It's a simple concept with complex implications, especially when it comes to our health and well-being.

It's common knowledge that negative emotions and stress can lead to physical ailments, but what if we flip the coin? Can positive thinking, then, lead to better health? Many experts would give a resounding "Yes" to that question. Harnessing the power of positive thinking can aid in stress management, an acknowledged factor in many health issues. But remember, it's not about blindly ignoring life's problems; it's about approaching hardships in a more positive and productive way. In a future chapter we will look at the super-power chemical that our brains naturally make to turn this concept into reality. The mind is a powerful tool, and understanding how to use it to positively influence your physical health can be a game-changer. So, the next time you're facing a health hurdle, remember it's not just about the physical. Your mind has a part to play, too, and learning how to effectively engage it could be your ticket to a healthier, happier you.

THE BATTLE WITH WILLPOWER AND MOTIVATION

We've all found ourselves in this predicament – aware that we ought to exercise or eat nutritious food, yet we're seduced by the allure of the sofa and a bag of chips. What transpires within our minds when motivation fades? Dean Bokhari has exposed the common offenders, such as fear of failure, procrastination, ambiguity, or even depression (BetterHelp; Bokhari). How, then, might we recognize our motivation-drainers and conquer them?

Initially, scrutinize your temperament and habits. Are you evading exercise due to apprehension of judgment from others? Or perhaps you're daunted by the excess of options, unsure where to begin? Determining the root cause of your motivational troubles enables you to build a plan to address them directly (Bokhari, n.d.).

STRATEGIES TO CONQUER MOTIVATION DEFICITS

Seeking motivation is a natural endeavor when you have none! Many tactics can provide the boost you desperately need. The National Institute on Aging recommends establishing specific goals, acquiring an exercise companion, or rewarding yourself post-workout (National Institute on Aging, n.d.). An additional valuable tip involves breaking tasks into smaller, more digestible steps, rendering them less intimidating.

Suppose you've resolved to go to the gym three times a week. Rather than arriving unprepared, develop a plan detailing the exercises you want to get through each day. Consequently, a consistent blueprint will guide you, simplifying your pledge to your routine. If motivation escapes you still, consider enlisting the support of a friend or family member. Accountability partners can prove invaluable in maintaining commitment to your objectives.

Remember, Rome wasn't erected overnight, and neither is a wholesome lifestyle. Exercise patience and revel in even the most minute victories. Incremental progress is still progress.

INTRINSIC GRATIFICATION – ACCESSING THE INNER REWARD SYSTEM

Having touched upon motivation, let us now address rewards. Not indulging in a tub of ice cream post-workout (an enticing notion, indeed), but rather, your brain's internal reward mechanism. A complex neural network within our brains facilitates pleasure and satisfaction, largely attributable to a neurotrans-mitter known as *dopamine*.

This remarkable chemical is released during pleasurable experiences such as eating, socializing, or even falling in love. Dopamine is instrumental in motivating us to repeat these enjoyable activities, thereby playing a pivotal role in habit formation (Dana Foundation, n.d.).

How, then, do we harness dopamine's power to render exer-cise and healthy living more gratifying?

The answer lies in exploiting innate rewards – those derived from within, as opposed to external sources. Consider the feel-ings of accomplishment following a rigorous workout or the surge in self-esteem upon realizing your clothes fit better. Such intrinsic rewards can bolster motivation throughout your journey toward improved health.

To transform exercise and healthy decisions into innate rewards, concentrate on the immediate benefits, such as enhanced mood, increased energy, or the sheer delight of move-ment. Seek activities that genuinely appeal to you and consciously recognize the positive emotions they evoke.

The more we participate in intrinsically rewarding activities, the more dopamine our brains release, fortifying the neural pathways associated with these pursuits (Greater Good Science Center at UC Berkeley, n.d.). Over time, this process converts once-arduous exercises into pleasurable habits more likely to be sustained.

Establishing new habits may demand time and effort, but the rewards are worthwhile. Envision a life where you eagerly anticipate workouts and relish making healthy choices.

Ah, the intrinsic rewards! Now that we've had our fill of those intellectual hors d'oeuvres, let's stroll into another room of this cerebral party: the growth mindset. Carol Dweck, a woman with enough brainpower to light up a small village, cooked up this tantalizing idea that suggests our minds and skills can be buffed and polished with a hearty dose of grit, tenacity, and an insatiable appetite for learning (Dweck, 2016).

Imagine, if you will, a fixed mindset: a dreary state in which people assume their talents are as immovable as the Sphinx, stubbornly resistant to change. But those with a growth mindset, those lively souls, eagerly embrace challenges, taste the nectar of feedback, and soldier on despite the occasional potholes – all crucial elements for a spiffier, healthier existence (*Psychology Today*, n.d.).

Now, how does this growth mindset get into your wellness struggle? Like a custom-tailored suit! Embracing this perspective enables you to invest the requisite effort to effect enduring changes in your life, encompassing both physical fitness and overall well-being.

With unwavering faith in your capacity to change and adapt, you'll be more inclined to exert yourself during workouts, experiment with novel nutritious recipes, and remain dedicated to your objectives, even in challenging times.

To nurture this growth mindset, embrace mistakes as learning opportunities, and keep in mind that progress – rather than perfection – is the true *pièce de résistance*. Surround yourself with positive influences, and always remember: each minuscule step you take moves you closer to the healthier, more joyful life you so richly deserve.

ACTIVITIES TO CULTIVATE MOTIVATION AND MINDSET SHIFTS

Arm yourself with your workbook or journal – it's time for introspective contemplation. Begin by asking yourself: "What's preventing me from realizing my health and fitness objectives?" Be frank, and don't hesitate to delve deep. Is the prospect of initiating a new workout regimen daunting? Is self-doubt creeping in, convincing you that you're incapable of change? By pinpointing the specific obstacles hampering your motivation, you'll be better prepared to confront them directly.

IDENTIFYING PERSONAL REASONS FOR WANING MOTIVATION

Let's be candid. We all experience days when summoning the motivation to engage in activities we know are beneficial proves challenging. The first step in overcoming this motivational deficit is identifying the genuine reasons behind it.

Here are several activities to help you detect your motivational hurdles:

- *Contemplate past experiences:* Spend a few moments reflecting on instances when you lacked motivation. Was it due to fatigue, stress, or feeling overwhelmed? Or was it because you didn't witness immediate results or doubted your ability to achieve your goals? Jot down your thoughts and search for patterns that may be contributing to your diminished motivation.

- *Evaluate your priorities:* Occasionally, we lose motivation because our objectives don't align with our true values and priorities. List your top five priorities in life, then examine whether your health and fitness goals support these priorities. If they don't, consider reassessing your goals to ensure they align with what genuinely matters to you.
- *Inspect your environment:* Your surroundings can significantly influence your motivation levels. Consider the people, places, and situations that may be sapping your energy or discouraging you from pursuing your goals. Identifying these external factors can help you implement necessary changes to foster a more supportive environment for your health (Bokhari, n.d.).

PROMOTING INTRINSIC REWARDS FOR MOTIVATION

Intrinsic rewards originate from within, such as the gratification of attaining a goal or the sense of accomplishment arising from surmounting a challenge. By focusing on intrinsic rewards, you can access your inner motivation and render healthy choices more pleasurable.

Here are some suggestions to help you foster intrinsic rewards for motivation:

- *Set significant, personal goals:* Rather than concentrating on external rewards (e.g., shedding weight to impress others), establish goals that are personally meaningful and aligned with your values. This might include enhancing your overall health to have more energy for your family or achieving a fitness milestone to demonstrate to yourself that you're capable of accomplishing great feats.

- *Maintain a progress journal:* Documenting your efforts can help you recognize your progress and celebrate small victories along the way. Record your achievements, challenges, and reflections in a journal, and review it regularly to remind yourself of the progress you're making.

- *Practice mindfulness:* Incorporating mindfulness techniques, such as meditation or deep breathing exercises, can help you remain present and fully appreciate the positive feelings and emotions stemming from engaging in healthy activities. By being more conscious of these intrinsic rewards, you're more likely to develop genuine enjoyment on your trip to good health (Greater Good Science Center at UC Berkeley, n.d.).

CULTIVATING A GROWTH MINDSET: YOUR PERSONAL ROADMAP TO SUCCESS

Believing that grit and persistence can refine one's intellect and prowess is at the core of a growth mindset. Embracing this philosophy can propel you past barriers, glean wisdom from setbacks, and fuel an unyielding quest for self-betterment.

Consider these savvy tactics to feed your growth mindset:

- *Embrace the challenge*: Welcome demanding tasks or situations as gateways to enlightenment and personal development. When faced with adversity, remind yourself it's an opportunity to sharpen your skills and fortify your resilience.
- *Treasure failure:* Missteps are inevitable companions on any voyage, but they're also priceless tutors. Should you stumble, pause to dissect the mishap, extract the lessons, and strategize your next move.
- *Swap negative musings for heartening declarations:* Our thoughts wield considerable power over our disposition and drive. Be intentional in substituting self-defeating chatter with resilient mantras that boost your faith in your capacity to evolve and excel.
- *Pursue guidance and friendship*: Engulf yourself in a supportive community who cheers on your growth and offers insightful critiques. Be it friends, kin, or professional mentors, actively solicit their wisdom and employ their suggestions for your personal advancement.
- *Relish the journey, not solely the destination*: To adopt a growth mindset is to cherish the odyssey as much as the final prize. Rather than fixating on goal attainment, savor each stride and celebrate incremental progress, ensuring motivation and an unwavering dedication to self-improvement.

By embracing these endeavors, you'll be on the fast track to nurturing motivation and adopting a growth mindset. Remember, wielding the formidable power of your mind is paramount to achieving lasting transformation. Pinpoint personal triggers of dwindling motivation, establish innate rewards, and deploy strategies to foster a growth mindset, thus laying the groundwork for a more vital and contented existence.

Bear in mind, metamorphosis isn't an overnight affair. It demands time, tenacity, and devotion to reshape your outlook and forge new habits. Be easy on yourself, and keep in mind that every small advancement propels you closer to your aspirations.

KEY TAKEAWAYS

1. Your mind plays a crucial role in your motivation levels, making it essential to address mental barriers to achieve your health and fitness goals.
2. By focusing on intrinsic rewards, you can turn healthy choices into enjoyable habits that stick.
3. Embracing a growth mindset empowers you to overcome challenges, learn from setbacks, and stay committed to personal improvement.
4. Identifying personal causes of lacking motivation and developing strategies to address them can lead to lasting change.
5. Surrounding yourself with positive in influences and shifting your perspective can help you break free from self-imposed limitations and make significant progress.

FINAL THOUGHTS

So, which person are you – the one who needs a gentle nudge or one who requires a more assertive push to start moving? No matter your answer, it's evident that overcoming mental barriers and tapping into the power of your mind is crucial for achieving lasting change.

You've delved into the power of your mind, pinpointed potential motivation obstacles, and begun nurturing a growth mindset. Now, it's time to take control of your life and make those positive changes you've been envisioning. Remember, the journey to a healthier, happier you originates with the first step. So, embrace your newfound knowledge, show yourself kindness along the way, and get ready to transform your life, one healthy choice at a time. The world is your oyster – conquer it!

As we proceed to the next chapter, we'll dive even deeper into the realm of mindset and discover how to break free from the chains of self-imposed limitations. Are you prepared to harness the power of your mind and leave those pesky excuses behind? Make it happen!

4

DOPAMINE – THE POWERHOUSE UNLOCKED

U nraveling the mysterious power of dopamine – that's the gist of this literary masterpiece. My goal is to reveal ideas and strategies that enable success in health, fitness, and longevity. Once achieved, the objective is to maintain this newfound stamina. The same principle applies to success in business: participate in productive practices and continue to reap the benefits. Success is realistic, with a bit of persistence. Inside your head and heart, this is an immeasurable pursuit, you will never get to the final destination, but the journey toward that mysterious and ultimate destination of good health, that is what we live for.

A word of caution: focusing only on the end goal is a risky struggle. Should your focus stay only on the fruits of your labor, motivation may decrease. Living continually at peak levels is unsustainable. In the pursuit of impressive achievements, dopamine may retreat, dipping below baseline levels and leaving motivation in the dust. Reclaiming those once-dizzying heights becomes an increasingly difficult task. The key, then, is to relish the voyage, embracing the triumphs and experiences along the way. This approach allows us to tap into the fascinating power of dopamine and harness its potential.

Has your motivation ever vanished, leaving you lost? Well, you are in good company. There is a method to "hack" the brain, rekindling the fire of motivation and drive. Say hello to dopamine, the cerebral "happy drug" accessible to one and all. By manipulating our inborn dopamine levels, we can persuade our brain into embracing change (health, fitness, etc.) as a most mouthwatering treat. Your brain will, no doubt, be eternally grateful.

In this chapter, I will show some of the hidden secrets of dopamine, revealing how this euphoria-inducing compound can invigorate your pursuit for success.

UNDERSTANDING DOPAMINE

Before we dive into the world of dopamine hacking, let's first understand what dopamine actually is. Remember, this is a simplified explanation because the actual processes in the brain are much more complex and involve many more steps and dynamics. But hopefully, this gives you a clearer picture of how things work.

Alright, let's think about this in the way you might think about baking a cake. When you bake, you start with raw ingredients that aren't very appealing on their own - flour, sugar, raw eggs. But when you combine them in the right way and put them through a process (baking), you get a delicious cake.

In our brain, we also have raw ingredients and processes that produce something we want, for example motivation.

Dopamine is one of these raw ingredients, like flour in your cake. It's a type of chemical that our brain cells, or neurons, use to communicate with each other, that's why neuroscientists call it a neuromodulator, and it plays a big part in how we feel pleasure and reward.

Now, you can't make a cake with just flour and in the same way, your brain can't make motivation with just dopamine. It needs to go through a process, and that's where norepinephrine and epinephrine (also known as adrenaline) come in. These are like the eggs and sugar in your cake.

There's an enzyme in your brain (kind of like a tiny molecular chef) called dopamine-beta-hydroxylase that takes dopamine and converts it into norepinephrine. Then, another enzyme called phenylethanolamine-N-methyltransferase takes norepinephrine and turns it into epinephrine or adrenaline. I hope I haven't lost you, stick with it and I'll get off the scientist wagon.

So how does this turn into motivation? Well, adrenaline is often associated with our body's "fight or flight" response. It helps to focus our attention, quicken our heartbeat, and prepare our bodies for action. But, in less extreme circumstances, it can also help boost our drive and motivation to take on challenging tasks like doing a difficult workout. It's similar to the heat from the oven that transforms the batter into a cake.

So, if you're tackling a hard task, your brain decides to bake a motivation cake. It takes dopamine, converts it into norepinephrine and then into adrenaline, and voila! You've got that extra push to get things done. To keep the baking process running smoothly, your brain has to maintain a good balance of all these ingredients. Too much or too little can throw off the recipe, just like in baking. That's why taking care of our brain health, through things like sleep, exercise, and good nutrition, is so important. Dopamine's relationship to motivation is central and its release is not only tied to experiencing rewards but also the anticipation of them, powering our drive to pursue activities that are rewarding. It helps us remain attentive to our future goals by attaching pleasure to the pursuit of those goals and hopefully, to our ultimate achievement.

DOPAMINE AND THE INTRINSIC REWARD SYSTEM

As we discussed in the previous chapter, an intrinsic reward system is all about the satisfying vibes that come from within, rather than external factors like money, praise, or chocolate (though those are nice, too). And guess who's responsible for those internal rewards?

You got it – dopamine!

When you do something that aligns with your goals or values, your brain releases dopamine, giving you a little burst of happiness and satisfaction. This release of dopamine encourages you to keep pursuing those activities that make you feel good, creating a positive feedback loop that promotes motivation and success.

So, how does dopamine help with motivation and overall success?

It all comes down to that fantastic feeling you get when you do something good for yourself. When you experience that dopamine rush, it propels you to keep chasing that feeling, ultimately helping you stay motivated and achieve your goals. Research has shown that increasing dopamine levels can lead to improved focus, productivity, and even creativity – all key ingredients for success. In a nutshell, the more dopamine you have, the more motivated and successful you're likely to be (Leaders First, 2019).

HACKING DOPAMINE FOR MOTIVATION AND SUCCESS

Ever feel like you're stuck in a motivational rut? You know that annoying state where you're endlessly scrolling through social media instead of tackling that mess in the garage or hitting the gym? Well, it turns out that with a few simple tricks, you can hack your brain's dopamine system and turbocharge your motivation like never before (Mental Health Daily, 2015).

You see, dopamine is a bit like your brain's personal cheerleader, reminding you and encouraging you to act and pursue your goals, because your history of feeling energized and motivated holds a strong memory for you. But sometimes, it needs a little bump in the right direction. Here's where the fun part comes in: by understanding how dopamine works, you can give it that prod and get your motivation back on track.

SETTING AND ACHIEVING SMALL GOALS – STIMULATE DOPAMINE RELEASE

One of the most effective ways to hack your dopamine system is by setting and achieving small, manageable goals. You might think that accomplishing something tiny, like making your bed or drinking a glass of water, is no big deal. But when it comes to dopamine, even the smallest victory can make a world of difference. Think about it. Every time you achieve a goal, no matter how small, your brain rewards you with a surge of dopamine. This feel-good chemical makes you want to repeat the experience, which is why setting easily achievable goals can help jump-start your motivation (Harvard Business Review, 2016). So, how do you put this into practice? Start by breaking down your larger goals into smaller, more manageable tasks. For example, instead of vowing to "get fit," set a goal to walk for ten minutes every day. This simple, achievable task will not only make your overarching goal feel less daunting but also give you a daily dose of dopamine to keep your motivation levels high.

DOPAMINE DOESN'T JUDGE

Ah, the dopamine game. It's a little dance we do with our brains, seeking out those delightful bursts of pleasure from the tiniest accomplishments. Picture this: you complete some inane chore, or sip on a glass of water, and – voila! – a miniature celebration erupts in your noggin. You see, dopamine is no snob. It celebrates in the seemingly mundane as much as the grandiose.

Now, imagine we harness this power, using it to propel ourselves through life's more onerous tasks. The secret? Crafting minuscule goals, ripe for the plucking. And the *pièce de résistance*? Ensuring these goals are, in fact, more challenging than the task at hand.

Picture yourself, knee-deep in the world of sprinkler repair (why is it always plumbing that annoys us?). You're armed with tools, hunting rogue nozzles, and excavating your once-pristine lawn. What could possibly be more difficult than this endless task, you ask? Well, science suggests that an ice-cold plunge, or perhaps a frigid shower, will do the trick. It's hard to believe, I know, but trust me – I've tried it. Two minutes of shivering bliss, and your dopamine levels will soar, carrying you through a solid two to three hours of increased peak levels. A quicker means to this is a face plunge into a near frozen salad bowl of icy water. It should be pretty uncomfortable. Hold your breath, face in until you can't take any more (different for everyone), and the fix is in. Eleven minutes per week separated into two-to-three minutes of deliberate cold exposure.

So, how to apply this in our everyday lives? Simple: break those lofty ambitions into bite-sized morsels. Don't just "get fit" – commit to a daily ten-minute walk. These manageable tasks not only render your overarching goal less intimidating but also gift you with a steady stream of dopamine, fueling your motivation to keep striding forward. Now, off you go – and don't forget to pack a towel for that icy shower. Of course, remember to make it cold enough to be miserable and uncomfortable, but doable.

BUILDING MOMENTUM WITH EASY GOALS

You know what's better than achieving one goal? Achieving a whole bunch of them! Once you've mastered the art of setting and achieving small goals, it's time to build on your success and create some serious momentum.

Think of it like a snowball effect: each time you achieve a goal and experience that dopamine-fueled sense of accomplishment, you'll be more motivated to tackle the next task on your list. Over time, this momentum will make it easier to achieve increasingly ambitious goals. (Harvard Business Review, 2016).

To build momentum, try following these steps:

1. *Set a series of easy goals that relate to your larger objective.*
   Remember, the key here is to make these goals
   achievable and specific. For example, if your ultimate
   goal is to lose weight, start with something simple
   like cutting out sugary snacks or going for a daily
   walk.
2. *Establish a routine.* Consistency is key when it comes to
   building momentum, so try to work on your goals at
   the same time every day. This will help cement your
   new habits and make it easier to stick to your plan.
3. *Celebrate your successes.* Don't be shy about giving
   yourself a pat on the back when you achieve a goal.
   Each time you celebrate your accomplishments,
   you're reinforcing the positive feelings associated with
   dopamine, making it more likely that you'll continue
   to pursue your goals.
4. *Gradually increase the difficulty of your goals.* As you build
   momentum and become more comfortable with your
   new routine, you can start to challenge yourself with
   more ambitious goals. Just remember to keep them
   manageable and specific to ensure that you maintain
   your motivation.

By hacking this system and using it to your advantage, you
can unlock the secret to supercharged motivation and finally
achieve the success you've always dreamed of. It's time to start
chasing those goals.

ACTIVITIES TO ENHANCE MOTIVATION

The first step is understanding what makes your brain tick. For one week, keep a journal of when you feel that rush of happiness, satisfaction, or motivation. Was it after a delicious meal? A brisk walk outside? A heart-to-heart conversation with a friend? By tracking your dopamine triggers, you'll gain insights into how your brain releases this feel-good chemical and how you can optimize those moments for maximum motivation (Cleveland Clinic).

There are some basic activities you can do that cost next to nothing and are proven to increase the levels of dopamine in individuals.

- *Sunlight:* Spend some time outdoors.
- *Exercise*: Don't neglect this component, the returns go beyond dopamine levels.
- *Cold Showers*: Hey, the science in this case doesn't lie.
- *Establish and Seek Long Term Goals*: It's the journey, not the destination.
- *Sleep*: Get some, your body and brain are craving it.

ANALYZING CURRENT REWARDS SYSTEMS

Now that you've got a better understanding of your dopamine triggers, it's time to take a closer look at your current reward system (Healthfully, n.d.). Do you treat yourself to a slice of pizza after a long day? Or perhaps a cold beer or a cocktail as a reward for finishing a project? While these external rewards can certainly be enjoyable, they may not be the most effective way to hack your dopamine system. Identifying how you currently reward yourself will help you understand which aspects of your reward system are working for you and which areas could use some re-tuning.

CREATING A PERSONALIZED DOPAMINE-DRIVEN REWARD SYSTEM

With your dopamine triggers and current reward system in mind, it's time to create a personalized, dopamine-driven reward system that will keep you motivated and on track. Focus on incorporating activities that you know trigger dopamine release for you, and make sure your rewards align with your goals and values.

For example, if exercise is a known dopamine trigger for you, try rewarding yourself with a short workout session after completing a task, rather than indulging in junk food. By swapping out less productive rewards for dopamine-boosting activities, you'll create a powerful feedback loop that will keep you motivated and moving forward.

ADAPTING AND EVOLVING GOALS AS THEY BECOME HABITS

As you start to build momentum with your small daily goals, you may find that they eventually become habits – which is fantastic! However, to keep the dopamine flowing, it's important to adapt and evolve your goals as they become second nature.

Try adding a new twist to your daily routine or setting a slightly more challenging goal to keep things fresh and engaging. By continually pushing yourself to grow and change, you'll maintain that dopamine-driven motivation and continue to make progress toward your larger goals.

KEY TAKEAWAYS

1. Dopamine is a powerful brain chemical linked to happiness, motivation, and the intrinsic reward system.
2. Understanding how dopamine works can help boost motivation and drive to achieve personal goals.
3. Setting and achieving small, manageable goals can stimulate dopamine release and enhance motivation.
4. Building momentum by consistently working on goals and celebrating achievements further boosts dopamine levels and motivation.
5. Hacking the dopamine system can unlock the potential for greater success and personal growth.

FINAL THOUGHTS

By understanding the power of dopamine and how it can shape your motivation and drive, you've unlocked a new level of potential within yourself. Remember, you have the ability to harness your brain's natural chemistry to fuel your quest for success. Start with small, achievable goals, and let the snowball effect of dopamine-driven motivation propel you toward greatness.

As you continue on, don't forget to celebrate your accomplishments, and build on your successes. It's time to embrace the power of dopamine and unleash your full potential. So go ahead – take a deep breath, set your sights high, and chase those dreams with the newfound knowledge that you have the tools to succeed.

In the next chapter we'll explore how to break free from old habits and embrace change. So, keep this dopamine train rolling, and together, we'll overpower the old habits!

5

YOU'RE NOT OLD, YOUR HABITS ARE

Picture this: it's a lovely day, and you're all set to go for a run. But somehow, you end up on the sofa, watching your Alma Mater pound their opponent on the football field, munching on junk, and promising yourself you'll start exercising tomorrow. Sounds like something you've been through, right? We all have habits we'd love to get rid of, but it seems so hard to do. Why do we keep doing things we know aren't good for us? Well, buddy, our brains are messing with us, and dopamine is the sneaky troublemaker.

Before we dig into habits, let's chat about why it's important to break these annoying patterns. Imagine how much better life would be without unhealthy and unproductive habits holding us back. We'd be stronger, more energetic, and healthier overall. If you're ready to ditch the bad habits keeping you from your best life, let's see how dopamine plays a part in keeping these habits alive and what we can do to break the cycle.

DOPAMINE - A DOUBLE-EDGED CHEMICAL

In our previous discourse, we extolled the virtues of dopamine as a magnificent motivator, fueling our internal reward machinery. We uncovered how this wondrous molecule propels us toward our objectives, sharpens our focus, and even elevates our mood. Simply put, dopamine is akin to that fantastic friend who ceaselessly encourages and inspires you to reach your full potential.

However, dopamine's splendor has a flip side. Our gray matter remains indifferent to the moral implications of an activity when it comes to dopamine release. Consequently, when we indulge in detrimental habits that offer fleeting gratification, our brains reward us with dopamine, making it even more challenging to abstain (Into Action Recovery Centers, n.d.).

Consider our affinity for sweets: when we yield to temptation and savor a delectable treat, our brains dispense dopamine, enveloping us in delight. Regrettably, this fleeting pleasure only fuels our cravings, and soon we find ourselves reaching for yet another donut or slice of cake. It's a textbook illustration of dopamine entwined with vice.

How can we escape this vicious circle? Recognize that our brains are wired to seek pleasure, and when we engage in harmful habits that elicit dopamine, we inadvertently reinforce them. The initial step toward liberation is comprehending that we are neither feeble nor defective; our brains are simply excelling at their task.

One strategy for breaking the cycle involves identifying and understanding the triggers that prompt our vices. If stress propels you toward sugary indulgences, acknowledging this trigger empowers you to seek healthier alternatives. Rather than devouring that chocolate bar, opt for a brisk walk, deep breathing exercises, or a chat with a good friend. By substituting the detrimental habit with a more wholesome one, you continue to reap the dopamine rewards without the drawbacks.

Another crucial step is to exercise patience with yourself. Modifying entrenched habits demands time, effort, and tenacity. Setbacks are inevitable but remember that progress rarely follows a linear trajectory. Revel in your victories, no matter their size, and extract wisdom from your missteps. Keep in mind that continuing with the struggle is what yields enduring transformation.

Finally, cultivate a supportive network of friends and family who understand your goals and can assist you in staying on course. Sharing triumphs and tribulations with others makes the adventure more enjoyable and bolsters your odds of success. As social creatures, knowing we are not isolated in our actions makes a world of difference.

Thus, we arrive at the crux of dopamine's role in our unwholesome habits. By comprehending the science underpinning our actions, we can liberate ourselves from the shackles of vice and forge a healthier, more joyful, and invigorated existence. With perseverance, resolve, and a little assistance from our buddy dopamine, there's no ceiling to our accomplishments! Begin by pinpointing the habit loop, comprising a cue, a routine, and a reward. For example, stress may serve as your cue, inciting stress-eating, with the dopamine surge from savoring comfort foods as the reward. Discerning these elements aids in unraveling the entanglement and devising a blueprint for change.

Have you ever wondered why you can't resist that morning cup of coffee or why you always seem to check your phone the moment you wake up? The answer lies in the fascinating world of habits. From childhood to adulthood, our lives are a tapestry of habits, with some woven tightly and others hanging loosely by a thread.

How habits are formed throughout our lives

Habits form when we repeatedly engage in a behavior that brings us pleasure or relief, creating neural pathways in our brains that strengthen over time. This process, known as neuro-plasticity, allows our brains to adapt and change in response to our experiences (Verywell Mind, n.d.). As we continue to perform the behavior, these neural connections become more deeply ingrained, making the habit more and more automatic, like driving home from work without even thinking about the route. This automaticity is a testament to the brain's incredible efficiency, as it saves cognitive resources by offloading repetitive tasks to well-worn neural pathways.

However, this efficiency can also lead to some less-than-desirable habits if we're not careful. Think about it. When we first learn to tie our shoes, it requires a significant amount of mental effort and attention. But after doing it countless times, our brains develop a sort of autopilot, allowing us to tie our shoes without even thinking about it. The same principle applies to other habits, both good and bad. For example, reaching for a sugary snack when we're feeling stressed or lighting up a cigarette in response to certain social cues can become ingrained behaviors that our brains default to without conscious thought.

How habits are sustained

Our sneaky friend dopamine plays a starring role in habit sustainability. As we mentioned earlier, dopamine is responsible for that oh-so-satisfying reward we experience after engaging in a behavior. It's our brain's way of saying, "Hey, that was awesome! Let's do it again!" And because our brains are wired to seek out pleasure, we're naturally inclined to repeat behaviors that trigger that sweet, sweet dopamine release. However, not all habits are created equal, and some can have a more significant impact on our lives than others. For example, daily exercise can lead to increased energy, better mood, and overall improved health. On the other hand, binge-watching Netflix every night can lead to a sedentary lifestyle and a serious case of FOMO (fear of missing out) when your friends talk about their latest adventures.

THE PROCESS OF BREAKING HABITS

Breaking habits can feel like trying to solve a Rubik's cube blindfolded while riding a unicycle – challenging, to say the least. But fear not! With a little understanding of the science behind habits and a healthy dose of determination, it's entirely possible to break free from even the most stubborn of routines. The first step is to identify the habit loop, which consists of a cue, a routine, and a reward. For example, your cue might be stress, leading to the routine of stress-eating, and the reward is the dopamine release you get from indulging in your favorite comfort foods. By recognizing these elements, you can start to untangle the knot and create a plan for change.

DISMANTLING THE DOPAMINE DANCE TO OVERCOME FRUSTRATING HABITS

To shatter our undesirable routines, first decipher the triggers and rewards that entangle us. These triggers could be emotional states, particular situations, or specific moments in time. The reward, as we've previously discussed, often takes the form of a dopamine surge derived from indulging in the habit. To outsmart the dopamine dance, become a discerning detective of your own conduct. Be acutely aware of when and why you partake in these unhelpful habits. Jotting down observations in your workbook/journal can be invaluable. The more you comprehend the triggers and rewards behind your habits, the more equipped you'll be to effect enduring transformations.

UNEARTHING HEALTHIER AVENUES FOR YOUR DOPAMINE DESIRES

Armed with your newfound knowledge of triggers and rewards, it's time to seek out healthier methods for satisfying that dopamine craving. Rather than lighting up a cigarette when under duress, consider a spirited stroll or some deep, calming breaths. Both of these alternatives can still deliver that dopamine delight, while bestowing additional health advantages. Exercise creativity in your search for substitute activities – the secret lies in finding something genuinely pleasurable and sustainable over time. Though it may require some experimentation, perseverance will eventually lead you to discover the ideal match.

GENTLY REPLACING UNHEALTHY HABITS WITH SUPERIOR ALTERNATIVES

When saying goodbye to unfavorable habits, adopting a measured, gradual approach is crucial for success. Attempting to overhaul your entire existence in one fell swoop can be disastrous or, at the very least, leave you in a bad mood. Focus instead on incrementally substituting your unhealthy habits with loftier options.

Let's say you've discovered that ceaseless social media scrolling devours hours of your day and leaves you feeling depleted. Rather than going cold turkey, allocate specific times for perusing your accounts and progressively reduce the time spent on social media. Fill the void with more meaningful or pleasurable activities, such as reading a novel, calling a friend, or embarking on a new hobby. As you incorporate these subtle modifications, you'll begin to observe the favorable impact of your enhanced habits. Courtesy of dopamine, you'll start to crave these novel pursuits in place of your previous indulgences (*Time*, n.d.).

Bear in mind that breaking bad habits can be a life-long struggle, and your progress may meander rather than follow a direct path. Exercise patience and toast to minor victories along the way. By comprehending dopamine's role in habit formation and employing the principles we've explored, you can commence the process of reshaping your life for the better – one habit at a time. Embrace the challenge and, soon enough, you'll find yourself reveling in the delightful intricacies of your newly acquired, healthier routines. Keep your chin up and remember that change is a long road best savored with patience, persistence, and a touch of humor.

ACTIVITIES FOR OVERCOMING BAD HABITS AND ESTABLISHING BETTER ONES

In this section, we'll walk through a step-by-step guide for overcoming bad habits and replacing them with healthier choices. We'll explore practical techniques for identifying and understanding the reasons behind your habits, crafting effective replacement habits, and reflecting on your progress.

By following these activities, you'll be well on your way to transforming your life for the better.

1. *Pinpoint one bad habit to change:* The first step to breaking free from bad habits is to choose one habit you'd like to change. It's best to start small, and not tackle a deeply ingrained habit like smoking immediately. Instead, focus on something manageable, such as resisting the temptation of a candy bar during the afternoon slump or cutting back on social media browsing before bedtime.

2. *Investigate the habit's roots and benefits:* Delve deeper into the habit you've chosen to change. What drives this habit? Are you reaching for that candy bar because you're genuinely hungry, or are you seeking a temporary energy boost to get through the afternoon? Identifying the underlying causes and benefits of your habit will help you devise a successful replacement habit that addresses those needs.

3. *Develop a replacement habit and try it for a week:* Now that you've identified the reasons behind your bad habit, it's time to create a replacement habit that fulfills the same needs in a healthier way. If hunger drives your candy bar craving, try snacking on a piece of fruit or a handful of nuts instead. If you're seeking an energy boost, consider taking a brisk walk or doing a short workout. Implement your replacement habit for one week and observe its impact on your life.

4. *Reflect on your progress, setbacks, and potential improvements:* After a week, take some time to reflect on your progress. How many times did you revert to your old habit? How did the replacement habit make you feel? Use this information to refine your approach and make the replacement habit even more enticing. Remember to celebrate your victories and recognize the progress you've made, no matter how small.

KEY TAKEAWAYS

1. Habits, once established, can persist for a long time unless we actively work to change them.
2. Breaking and changing habits is challenging but crucial for replacing harmful behaviors with healthier ones.
3. Understanding the role of dopamine in habit formation can provide valuable insights for habit change.
4. Identifying the reasons behind a bad habit and creating a replacement habit are key steps in the process.

5. Reflecting on progress and celebrating wins, however small, can help maintain motivation and reinforce positive change.

FINAL THOUGHTS

Moving through life, change is a constant companion. Yet, we hold the power to direct that change, transforming it into a positive force in our lives. By comprehending the science behind our habits and leveraging the influence of dopamine, we can break the chains of old patterns and establish new, healthier habits that foster our well-being.

Encountering challenges is an inherent part of life, but with the appropriate mindset and resources, we can surmount these hurdles and emerge more resilient than ever. As you continue on your path toward positive aging, remember, you possess the power to rewire your mind, break the cycle of unhealthy habits, and seize the opportunities for growth and transformation.

6

ENGINEER YOUR PATH TO WELLNESS – MASTER YOUR HEALTH

E ver feel like growing older is a rickety old roller coaster ride? Overflowing with peaks and valleys, exhilarating chapters, and instances when all we want is to shut our eyes and wish it would all go away. There's a catch – getting off isn't an option, so, we might as well squeeze all we can out of it. And in case you didn't know, your psychological wellness as you age plays an increasing critical role in how much you enjoy this wild experience.

In this chapter, we'll explore the cooperative dance between your mental and physical health as you age, the impact of happiness on your longevity, and the value of purposefully guiding your mind for widespread well-being.

THE TANGLED TANGO OF MENTAL AND PHYSICAL HEALTH

I cannot overemphasize the elaborate entanglement between our mental state and our physical well-being. Tell me you're not acquainted with "it-has-been-one-of-those-days" kind of day. Fumbling with coffee, ensnared in traffic congestion, inadvertently erasing vital information, or leaving important paperwork on the counter – it's evident how mental wellness shapes our physical state. Conversely, an optimistic disposition can invigorate and propel us toward dealing with the day as it unravels around us with the knowledge that, soon, it will be over. The intertwined nature of mental and our physical health is indisputable; envision them as a flawlessly synchronized duo.

Mental health considerably sways our physical health. Tension and apprehension can materialize as migraines, stomach cramps, or cardiac flutters. Furthermore, miserable moods might lure us into harmful habits like overindulging, tobacco use, or excessive beverages. Persistent stress may also deplete our immune defenses, elevating susceptibility to illnesses and afflictions – which is an undesirable outcome in our twilight years.

On the flip side, physical health assumes a part in our mental equilibrium. Sedentary routines correlate with heightened depression risk, whereas consistent exercise can elevate spirits and mitigate stress. Additionally, certain physical ailments, such as chronic discomfort, cardiac issues, or diabetes, can exacerbate despondency and anxiety (Ontario CMHA, n.d.).

Attaining consonance between mental and physical health may feel akin to traversing a tightrope, but it's vital for aging with confidence. If you're physically robust but perpetually strained or disheartened, you're not genuinely savoring life to the fullest. Similarly, mental satisfaction coupled with subpar physical health deprives you of an extended, gratifying existence.

DECODING YOUR MIND AND MENTAL HEALTH – THE BONUSES

Who wouldn't yearn to unleash their mind's untapped capacity for a more blissful, happy, and enriched life? Concentrating on mental health can empower you to precisely do that. So, let's look at unveiling the perks of mental flourishing – From Life Enrichment to Potential Life Extension:

1. *Elevating the Quality of Life* Adeptly tending to one's mind and mental wellness has a magnificent ripple effect on your life's tapestry. Indulge in self-nourishment, express gratitude, and foster an ever-evolving mindset to invigorate your mood, personal connections, and general contentment. Moreover, a fortified psyche lends a helping hand in stress management and sailing through life's unavoidable trials.

2. *Unfurling the Secrets of Longevity* Craving the fountain of youth? Happiness is the master key. A renowned Harvard study uncovered that happy souls bask in lengthier, healthier lives (Harvard Health Publishing, 2019). By feeding mental well-being, you not only elevate daily moments but could also tack on precious years to your life – and that's something to smile about!

3. *Fortifying Physical Vigor* The undeniable bond between mental and physical wellness is one to behold. A sound mind inspires indulgence in activities that boost bodily health, like exercise, nourishing food, and adequate sleep. Moreover, a tenacious mental state can hasten recovery from sickness or injury and enhance our immune system capabilities. Essentially, a healthy and hearty mind lays the groundwork for a thriving physique – which is an objective worth chasing!

CHALLENGING THE TRIALS OF AGING – SOME NIFTY POINTERS

Let's rummage around and dig into the realm of realistic tips for conquering the trials of aging. Armed with a mindset and well-established systems, you can sail gracefully through aging, thriving along the way.

First off, think about feeding a sharpened mind and solid mental health through your social connections and engaging in activities you enjoy. I golf, so it not only keeps my mental health intact (that's a joke), but I also keep company with some awesome friends who help me maintain a sense of humor. (They're actually laughing at me and my game.)

Second, let's examine physical undertakings that support mental well-being. Exercise presents benefits not only upon your physique but also your psyche. Consistent physical exertion eases depression and anxiety symptoms, sharpens cognitive faculties, and elevates self-worth. As you advance in age, opt for gratifying activities that align with your physical prowess, like walking, swimming, yoga, or maybe even dancing. The objective is to unearth activities that spark joy and reinforce your mental health.

Last, let's tackle unearthing purpose and significance as we age. Our functions and obligations may evolve with time, presenting challenges in discovering purpose and meaning. Yet, the opportunity to make impactful contributions to your loved ones, your sphere of friends, and the world at large endures. Engaging in volunteer work, mentorship of co-workers, teenagers who would cherish attention from a caring adult, or lifelong learning can rekindle your sense of purpose and preserve an upbeat outlook.

Take my pal Bob, for instance, who devotes time each week to a local food bank – his aura has transformed, radiating happiness and life satisfaction. Even while employed, the workplace offers a great setting for social interaction. Change is hard, there is no getting around that reality, but studies reveal that as we age and can hold on to a robust sense of purpose, retain cognitive abilities and relish exceptional mental health. So, dare to venture into fresh interests – you never know where they might lead you!

A RENAISSANCE OF AGING – THE EVERYDAY TOOLKIT THAT MASTERS MIDLIFE ADVENTURE

Aging is an inevitable process we all experience, and it's not without its hurdles. Nonetheless, equipped with the right mindset and strategies, you can confront these challenges head-on and continue to prosper as you age. In this section, we'll provide tips for managing the mental and physical challenges that often accompany aging, from fostering mental health through social connections and activities to unearthing purpose and meaning in life.

FORTIFYING MENTAL HEALTH THROUGH ENGAGING ACTIVITIES AND SOCIAL BONDS

One of the most powerful ways to maintain a sharp mind and robust mental health as you age is by nurturing social connections and immersing yourself in enjoyable activities. Pursuing hobbies, volunteering, or joining clubs can reinforce a sense of purpose and generate opportunities for valuable social interactions.

Research indicates that older adults with solid social connections have lower risks of cognitive decline, depression, and even mortality (Innerbody Research, n.d.). So, seize the day and embrace life's myriad experiences!

PHYSICAL PURSUITS THAT ENHANCE MENTAL WELL-BEING

Exercise isn't merely a boon for your body – it's also vital for your mind. Regular physical activity offers an excess of mental health advantages, including alleviated depression and anxiety symptoms, sharpened cognitive function, and heightened self-esteem (American Psychological Association, 2020).

As you advance in years, it's essential to discover activities that are both pleasurable and appropriate for your physical capabilities. These might encompass walking, swimming, yoga, or even dancing. Remember, the goal is not to be the fastest or strongest, but to find pursuits that bring joy and bolster your mental health.

UNEARTHING CONTINUED PURPOSE AND SIGNIFICANCE

As the years go by, our roles and responsibilities often evolve, and finding a sense of purpose and meaning in life can become challenging. If you are gainfully employed or run a business, you have no confusion about your purpose. Nonetheless, it's crucial to recognize that you can make meaningful contributions to your family, co-workers, or employees or to the ever-shrinking world.

Engaging in volunteer work, mentoring younger co-workers, or pursuing lifelong learning opportunities can reignite your sense of purpose and help you maintain a positive perspective on life. Studies suggest that adults with a robust sense of purpose are more likely to preserve their cognitive abilities and enjoy better overall mental health. So, be bold in exploring new passions and interests – you never know what exciting paths they may reveal!

THE MENTAL HEALTH PERKS OF EXERCISE AND PHYSICAL ACTIVITY

We're all familiar with the mantra: exercise is good for you. But did you know the benefits extend beyond your physical well-being? Indeed, exercise and physical activity also wield a profound influence on mental health. So, let's don those sneakers and delve into the marvelous realm of mood-lifting, stress-relieving, and mind-enhancing exercise!

UPLIFTING MOOD AND SELF-WORTH

Picture this: you've just completed a demanding workout and feel on top of the world, despite the exhaustion and sweat. You're not alone – research has demonstrated that regular exercise can significantly enhance mood and self-esteem.

As it turns out, engaging in physical activity prompts your body to release endorphins, those delightful chemicals responsible for a natural high (American Psychological Association, 2020). So, when the blues strike, remember that exercise acts as nature's very own mood booster, sans side effects.

ALLEVIATING STRESS AND ANXIETY

Life, as we know, can be incredibly stressful. But before you succumb to the allure of comfort food or a blanket cocoon, consider taking a jog or hitting the gym. Exercise has been shown to alleviate stress and anxiety by decreasing cortisol levels and increasing the production of chemicals that combat these negative emotions. Moreover, concentrating on your workout can distract you from your concerns, offering a much-needed mental reprieve. So, go ahead and sweat out that stress – your mind will surely be grateful.

CULTIVATING A POWERFUL MIND AND ENDURING MEMORIES

Who wouldn't desire a more agile mind and enhanced memory? Fortunately, exercise has been proven to boost cognitive function and memory across all ages. Engaging in physical activity nourishes your brain with ample oxygen and essential nutrients, fostering the growth of new neurons and bolstering overall brain health.

Moreover, exercise is associated with the production of a protein called BDNF, crucial for learning, memory, and cerebral function. So, if you're seeking to maintain your brain in prime condition, remember to incorporate regular workouts into your schedule, both mental and physical.

MINDFUL ENDEAVORS – DAILY PURSUITS FOR A JOYFUL, VIBRANT LIFE

Having delved into the remarkable benefits of exercise and physical activity on mental health, it's time to apply this newfound knowledge. Below are a few activities to encourage reflection on your personal trip and pinpoint daily pursuits that foster happiness and well-being.

REVISITING PERSONAL FEARS AND THEIR TRANSFORMATION

Take a moment to reflect on the three most significant fears you noted in your journal from Chapter 1. How do you perceive these fears now? Have they evolved or diminished as you've gained insight into the power of your mind and the importance of mental and physical health? Contemplate your progress and consider strategies for continuing to confront these fears while striving for a joyful, healthier future.

IDENTIFYING DAILY PURSUITS THAT ENCOURAGE HAPPINESS AND HOLISTIC WELL-BEING

Happiness is a vital component of our overall health and well-being, and integrating activities that spark joy into our daily lives can profoundly impact our mental and physical health. Jot down two things that bring you immense happiness and can be done every day. These might be as simple as taking a stroll, spending time with loved ones, or indulging in a hobby. By enhancing your overall happiness, you'll be well on your way to a healthier, more vibrant life.

KEY TAKEAWAYS

1. Mental and physical health are interconnected and can directly affect each other.
2. Hacking your mind and prioritizing your mental health can lead to improved quality of life, increased longevity, and enhanced physical health.
3. Aging presents challenges, but staying socially connected, engaging in physical activity, and finding purpose and meaning in life can help overcome these obstacles.
4. Exercise has numerous mental health benefits, including boosting mood, reducing stress and anxiety, and enhancing cognitive function and memory.
5. Incorporating activities that bring happiness into daily life can have a profound impact on overall health and well-being.

FINAL THOUGHTS

Aging can indeed be challenging, but always remember that we hold the power to shape our experiences. By giving equal importance to our mental and physical health, we can elevate our quality of life, potentially live longer, and boost our overall well-being. It's time to conquer our minds and tackle the challenges that aging brings.

The good news is that it's never too late to make positive changes in our lives. We can maintain social connections, stay active, find purpose, and infuse our daily routines with activities that bring us happiness. By doing so, we can craft a life that's fulfilling, dynamic, and enjoyable.

So, seize control of your mind and body and make the most of this thrilling ride. Focus on the things that bring us joy and give priority to our mental and physical health. By doing this, we can age gracefully, stay healthy, and savor every moment of this amazing journey.

In the upcoming chapter, we'll dig into the impact of physical activity on the aging process, the perks of various exercises, and practical tips for staying active as we grow older.

7

IN PURSUIT OF MOTION – REKINDLING THE PLEASURE OF MOBILITY

Ah, the good old days – when sprinting across the playground and hitting baseballs out of the park came naturally. Those carefree moments may be in the rearview mirror, but there's still a world of possibility waiting for you! The secret to unlocking a healthier, more fulfilling life lies in embracing exercise, fitness, and strength training as we move through the years.

TAKING STOCK OF YOUR CURRENT FITNESS REGIME

Before embarking on this new adventure, it's time for some soul-searching. Take a moment to reflect: What does your current exercise routine look like? Are you a neighborhood wanderer, a garage gym aficionado, or a living room yogi? Or perhaps you're more of a couch surfer, binging the latest series with an occasional snack run? Honesty is paramount here, as this self-assessment will illuminate the path toward improvement.

With your present fitness habits in mind, let's compare them to the recommended standards for men over 50. The Physical Activity Guidelines for Americans suggest at least 150 minutes of moderate-intensity aerobic activity or 75 minutes of vigorous-intensity aerobic activity per week, combined with muscle-strengthening activities on two or more days per week. Some experts even advocate for three or four sessions of weightlifting! (Centers for Disease Control and Prevention, n.d.)

Are you hitting these benchmarks, or is there room to grow?

It's essential to take ownership of your exercise habits because, ultimately, you're the one steering the ship. If you find yourself falling short of these guidelines, remember, they're guidelines, not gospel, and you can always change course. However, being realistic about your starting point is crucial. Temporary solace in denial won't propel you toward lasting health and well-being.

So, take a deep breath and scrutinize your current exercise routine (or lack thereof). Ask yourself: Am I doing enough to preserve my health and vitality as I age? Or am I passively allowing my body to decline? There's no judgment here – we're all navigating different waters. But now is the time to take the helm and make the necessary adjustments to ensure you're not just surviving, but flourishing as you mature.

As the great philosopher Socrates once proclaimed, "The unexamined life is not worth living." In our context, the unexamined exercise routine is not worth preserving. So, let's craft a plan to get you moving, invigorated, and ready to embrace the best version of yourself.

HERE'S A RECOMMENDED EXERCISE ROUTINE

1. *Warm-up*: Start with a five-to-ten-minute warm-up, including light aerobic activity such as marching in place or walking, to increase your heart rate and warm up your muscles.
2. *Aerobic exercise*: Aim for at least 150 minutes of moderate-intensity aerobic activity or 75 minutes of vigorous-intensity aerobic activity per week. Some options include:
3. Brisk walking
4. Swimming
5. Cycling
6. Dancing
7. Hiking
8. Water aerobics
9. Tennis or pickleball
10. *Strength training*: Incorporate strength training exercises at least two days per week, targeting all major muscle groups. Examples include:
11. Bodyweight exercises (push-ups, squats, lunges, etc.)
12. Weightlifting (dumbbells, barbells, or kettlebells)
13. Resistance bands
14. Machine exercises at a gym
15. *Flexibility and balance*: Add flexibility and balance exercises to your routine two-to-three times per week. These exercises can help improve posture,

prevent injuries, and increase overall mobility. Some options are:

16. Yoga
17. Pilates
18. Tai Chi
19. Stretching routines (e.g., hamstring stretches, calf stretches, shoulder stretches)
20. *Cool-down*: Finish your workout with a five-to-ten-minute cool-down, including light aerobic activity and stretching to gradually lower your heart rate and help prevent muscle soreness.

To truly optimize your fitness routine, you'll want to incorporate a mix of aerobic exercise, strength training, and flexibility work. Aerobic exercises, like brisk walking, swimming, or dancing, get your heart pumping and improve cardiovascular health. Strength training exercises, such as lifting weights, doing push-ups, or using resistance bands, help build and maintain muscle mass, which becomes increasingly important as we age. And finally, flexibility exercises, like yoga or stretching, can help maintain range of motion and prevent injury.

Think of it as a well-rounded fitness buffet. You wouldn't want to fill your plate with just one type of food, right? Same goes for your exercise routine. Mix it up to keep things interesting and ensure you're reaping all the benefits that physical activity has to offer. Exercise isn't just about looking good in a swimsuit (though, hey, that's a nice bonus).

Regular physical activity plays a crucial role in maintaining overall health and well-being as we age. Exercise can help reduce the risk of chronic diseases like heart disease, diabetes, and some cancers, improve mental health, and even help you live longer. It's like a magical elixir that keeps you feeling young and spry, even as the calendar pages keep turning. So, if you're not already on the exercise bandwagon, it's time to hop on board.

Remember to listen to your body, and if you are anything like me, that shouldn't be an issue. My body doesn't offer up polite little whispers to "reel it in just a bit" – it usually screams and demands I shut it down, NOW! So, modify exercises as needed to accommodate any existing health conditions or physical limitations and respectfully tell your body, its days of telling you what you can and can't do are nearly over. It's always a good idea to consult with your healthcare provider before starting a new exercise routine, especially if you have any chronic health conditions or concerns. Also, consider working with a certified personal trainer or fitness professional who can help you create a tailored exercise plan that meets your specific needs and goals.

EXERCISE OPTIONS FOR MEN OF OUR STATURE

Now that you're aware of the exercise categories to incorporate into your routine, it's time to delve into specifics. The secret to success lies in identifying workouts and exercises tailored to your unique needs and abilities. You're no longer in your twenties, so there's no need to compete with CrossFit enthusiasts at the gym. Instead, concentrate on finding exercises suited to you and your particular circumstances.

Numerous workouts and exercises are ideal for mature men, including low-impact activities like swimming or cycling, strength training exercises using your body weight, and balance exercises to help prevent falls. The key is to pay attention to your body and adapt exercises as necessary to accommodate any limitations or health concerns.

For instance, if traditional push-ups are too demanding, try doing them against a wall or with your hands on an elevated surface like a countertop. If you have trouble with balance, consider using a chair or wall for support during exercises like lunges or squats. Remember, there's no disgrace in adapting exercises to meet your needs. The objective is to remain active and healthy, not to demonstrate that you can still bench press a substantial weight.

As you commence your new fitness trek, think about seeking professional assistance. A personal trainer or fitness instructor can help you devise a safe and effective workout plan tailored to your individual needs, objectives, and limitations. Moreover, they can offer guidance on proper form and technique to reduce the risk of injury. And let's be honest, having someone hold you accountable can make a significant difference when motivation begins to fade.

If a personal trainer isn't a feasible option, don't worry. Numerous other resources are available to assist you in navigating the fitness world. Many community centers and gyms offer exercise classes specifically designed for older adults, and there's no lack of workout videos and apps catering to a more mature audience. Just ensure that you consult with your doctor before starting any new exercise routine, particularly if you have any pre-existing health conditions or concerns.

Remaining active and maintaining a well-rounded fitness routine is essential for men over 50 who wish to age gracefully and preserve their overall health and well-being. By evaluating your current activity level, adhering to the recommended guidelines for physical activity, and customizing workouts to suit your individual needs and abilities, you'll be on the path to a healthier, more vibrant future. So, tie up those sneakers, brush off that old gym bag, and let's get moving!

YOUR FITNESS

Initiating your fitness project can be intimidating, particularly as you age. However, with the appropriate tactics and mindset, you can conquer any obstacles and make physical activity a fundamental part of your daily life. Taking the initial step is the hardest part of any endeavor. Armed with the proper strategies and mindset, you can surmount any obstacles and seamlessly incorporate physical activity into your daily life.

In this section, I'll cover tips for increasing your exercise, cultivating new habits, and the significance of consistency in achieving success.

Approaches for Boosting Your Exercise and Accomplishing Your Goals

So, you've evaluated your current activity level and recognized that it's time to step up your game. Great! But where do you start? I have foolproof approaches to help you not only enhance your exercise but also crush those fitness goals like the unstoppable, age-defying rockstar you are.

First and foremost, establish realistic and attainable goals. It may be tempting to aim for a marathon next month, but it's crucial to start with smaller, more manageable objectives. This could involve taking a 30-minute walk daily, swimming laps at the local pool, or trying a new exercise class. Remember, nothing of value is ever built in a day, and your new exercise routine won't be either.

Another vital strategy is to make a plan and adhere to it. You must be a coaching badass! Do not allow the weak and easily distracted part of you try to dismantle what you've decided to attain. Schedule your workouts as you would any other appointment or obligation. This helps you stay organized and focused while making it harder to justify skipping a workout. Pro tip: Attempt to schedule your exercise during the time of day when you feel most energetic and motivated.

INTEGRATING NEW EXERCISE HABITS INTO YOUR DAILY ROUTINE

We all know that old habits die hard, particularly when it comes to incorporating new exercise routines into our daily lives. However, with a touch of ingenuity and persistence, you can smoothly blend these healthy habits into your everyday life.

Begin by identifying opportunities to be more active throughout your day. This could mean using the stairs instead of the elevator, parking further from the grocery store entrance, or walking to a nearby coffee shop during your lunch break. The more you can incorporate physical activity into your day, the easier it becomes to sustain your new exercise habits.

Another method to integrate new exercise habits is by discovering activities you genuinely enjoy. If the idea of running on a treadmill sounds dreadful, consider trying something more appealing, like dancing, yoga, or even a team sport. When you find an activity you love, exercise feels less like a chore and more like an enjoyable, rewarding part of your day.

THE SIGNIFICANCE OF CONSISTENCY AND ACCOUNTABILITY IN ACHIEVING SUCCESS

Consistency is crucial when it comes to building and maintaining new exercise habits. By adhering to your routine and making exercise an indispensable part of your day, you'll begin to notice improvements in your fitness, energy levels, and overall well-being.

Accountability is another essential element of success. Whether it's teaming up with a workout buddy, employing a personal trainer, or joining a group class, having someone to be accountable can help keep you on track and motivated. Moreover, exercising with others can make the experience more enjoyable and social, which is always a bonus. When I first started, I gave my wife permission to challenge me (sometimes confront me) with both food and exercise choices. When eating better and exercise became part of my regular routine, I found I need fewer challenges.

STICKING TO YOUR TIMETABLE – HOLD YOURSELF ACCOUNTABLE

Tracking your progress and celebrating your achievements Tracking your progress is crucial for staying motivated and ensuring you're making progress toward your fitness goals. Create a simple log or use a fitness app to track your workouts, including the type, duration, and intensity of each activity. Regularly review your log to monitor your progress and adjust your routine if needed.

In addition to tracking your progress, make sure to applaud your achievements, no matter how small. Acknowledging your hard work and accomplishments helps build self-confidence and encourages you to keep pushing forward.

Evaluating your progress and adjusting your goals after three weeks

After three weeks, take some time to evaluate your progress. Have you achieved your goals? If so, congratulations! If not, don't be discouraged. Reflect on any challenges or obstacles you faced and consider how you can overcome them moving forward.

Use your evaluation to set new goals for the next three weeks, building on the progress you've already made. Remember to keep your goals realistic and achievable while still pushing yourself to make continuous improvements.

Staying engaged and committed to your fitness

The road to health is a lifelong battle, and staying engaged and committed is essential for long-term success. Keep experimenting with new activities and routines to keep things fresh and exciting, and seek out support from friends, family, or a fitness community to help you stay motivated and accountable.

Your fitness is unique to you, and you have the power to shape it however you'd like. Embrace the challenges, celebrate your achievements, and enjoy the process of becoming a healthier, more vibrant version of yourself. With dedication and perseverance, you'll be well on your way to a lifetime of fitness and well-being.

KEY TAKEAWAYS

1. Assessing your current activity level and being honest with yourself is crucial for making improvements.
2. Following the recommended guidelines for exercise for men over 50 can significantly impact overall health and well-being.
3. A balanced workout plan, tailored to individual needs and capabilities, is key to staying active and healthy as you age.
4. Kickstarting your fitness requires setting realistic goals, incorporating new habits into your daily routine, and maintaining consistency. Actively engaging in the activities provided can help you make lasting, positive changes in your routine and overall health.

FINAL THOUGHTS

As I conclude this chapter, always remember that it is never too late to begin your passage. Your age should never hinder your quest to improve your health and well-being. Regardless of your current stage in life, there is always an opportunity to take control of your body, build strength, and elevate your quality of life. If you have made it to about the halfway portion of this book, congratulations! If you started your journey and stopped, start again. Sometimes life gets in the way of doing all that we want. However, if there were one thing you don't want to give up on, it's your health.

So, go ahead, embrace the challenges, get the dopamine cranking again, and rejoice in the small triumphs along the way.

As you progress, bear in mind that you're not only adding years to your life but also infusing life into your years. Your future self will be grateful for the initial step you take today. Remain active, maintain your health, and continue moving forward.

Two adaptable exercises for us:

https://fitnessdrum.com/kettlebell-workout-for-over-50s/
https://www.livestrong.com/article/13721878-strength-train
ing-workout-over-50/

8

SOOTHING THE STORM OF PAIN –
YOUR PATH TO RELIEF

L et's face it: aches and pains can be a real pain in the...
well, you know where. We've all used those stiff knees or
sore shoulders as excuses to dodge exercise. However, exercise
might actually be a game-changer for managing arthritis! By
staying active, you can alleviate those annoying aches. In this
chapter, I'll guide you through the magic of arthritis management with exercise. It's time to ditch the excuses and discover
workouts that help your joints and overall health.

I know what you're thinking: "Exercise for arthritis? Seriously?" There is much research to back this up. Exercise can do
wonders for arthritis sufferers – not only easing pain but also
enhancing joint function, making daily tasks more doable.

Studies reveal that regular exercise can reduce joint pain,
boost strength, improve flexibility, and increase endurance, all
while helping you maintain a healthy weight (which is a plus
for those with arthritis).

So, let's talk about exercise for arthritis management. You might be wondering, "What kind of exercises should I try?" Great question! There's a variety of exercises that can help with arthritis, generally falling into three categories: aerobic, strengthening, and flexibility/balance exercises.

Aerobic exercises (aka "cardio") are activities that get your heart pumping and enhance overall fitness. They can help diminish inflammation and improve joint function. Some low-impact, arthritis-friendly aerobic exercises include walking, swimming, cycling, and even dancing (just save those break-dancing moves for another occasion).

Strengthening exercises, as the name implies, focus on building muscle strength. Stronger muscles better support your joints and reduce the strain on them, which can help ease pain. Arthritis-friendly strengthening exercises include resistance training with bands or light weights, bodyweight exercises like modified push-ups or squats, and even water-based exercises.

Lastly, flexibility, balance, and hip mobility exercises help maintain your range of motion and lower your risk of falls – super important for those with arthritis. Gentle stretching, yoga, and tai chi are fantastic ways to work on flexibility and balance, plus they can also help relieve stress and tension in your muscles and joints.

RECOMMENDATION FOR EXERCISES TO MANAGE ARTHRITIS

If you are ready to show arthritis pain who's boss, then read on. Let's explore exercise options tailored to help manage arthritis. In this section, we'll talk about different exercise types, like aerobic, strengthening, and flexibility exercises, and provide examples to help you craft a balanced, arthritis-friendly workout routine. Keep in mind that it's essential to find exercises that suit you and your unique situation, so be ready to experiment and discover what is most manageable for your body.

AEROBIC EXERCISES: PUMP UP YOUR HEART

Aerobic exercises play a vital role in managing arthritis. They help diminish inflammation, enhance joint function, and keep your heart in tip-top shape. For aerobic exercises, consider low-impact activities like walking, swimming, cycling, or dancing. Just make sure you're not attempting any complex dance moves during your warm-up, and always check with your doctor before starting a new exercise routine.

STRENGTHENING EXERCISES: MUSCLE POWER FOR JOINT SUPPORT

Strengthening exercises are equally important for arthritis management. Building robust muscles around your joints can help lessen pain and strain, making movement easier. Resistance training with bands or light weights, bodyweight exercises like modified push-ups or squats, and water-based exercises are all fantastic options for strengthening your muscles without aggravating your arthritis.

FLEXIBILITY AND BALANCE EXERCISES – STRETCH AND BALANCE IT OUT

Flexibility and balance exercises help maintain your range of motion, lower your risk of falls, and ease stress and tension in your muscles and joints. Gentle stretching, yoga, and tai chi are all excellent choices for working on flexibility and balance. Just steer clear of any extreme positions that could lead to a tumble!

EXAMPLES OF SPECIFIC EXERCISES FOR ARTHRITIS MANAGEMENT

Now that we've covered the types of exercises, let's get specific. Here are some examples of arthritis-friendly exercises for each category:

1. *Aerobic:* Walking, swimming, cycling, water aerobics, or dancing (but perhaps save the twerking for another time)
2. *Strengthening:* Resistance band exercises, seated leg extensions, seated bicep curls, modified push-ups, or wall squats
3. *Flexibility/Balance:* Gentle stretches, yoga poses like child's pose or tree pose, tai chi movements, or even practicing standing on one foot while holding onto a chair for support

TIPS AND TRICKS FOR STARTING AN EXERCISE ROUTINE WITH ARTHRITIS

Arthritis comes in many forms and severities, so it's important to choose exercises that are appropriate for your specific condition. Talk to your doctor about which activities are best for you, and always remember to start slow and gradually increase the intensity of your workouts (Cleveland Clinic, 2021).

When starting an exercise routine with arthritis, it's crucial to be patient with yourself. Begin with gentle exercises and gradually increase the intensity as your body adapts. Nothing of value happens overnight, and neither will your new arthritis-friendly exercise routine.

As you exercise, pay attention to how your body feels. If you experience pain or discomfort, it's essential to listen to your body and adjust your routine accordingly. Remember, you're exercising to manage your arthritis, not to win an Olympic gold medal. It's better to take it easy than to push yourself too hard and end up sidelined.

If you're unsure about where to start or want some extra guidance, consider working with a physical therapist, personal trainer, or exercise specialist experienced in arthritis management. They can help create a tailored exercise plan that caters to your specific needs and goals. Plus, having a professional in your corner can provide motivation and accountability to keep you on track.

THE POWER OF CONSISTENCY AND COMMITMENT

Commencing your arthritis exercise is just the beginning. To truly enjoy the benefits and improve your quality of life, commit to staying consistent with your routine.

In this section, I'll explore strategies for establishing a regular exercise schedule, staying motivated, and holding yourself accountable. I'll also discuss the importance of evaluating your progress and adjusting as needed.

DEVELOPING A REGULAR EXERCISE ROUTINE

Consistency is the key to managing arthritis through exercise. Make exercise a regular part of your daily routine, just like brushing your teeth or trimming your nose hairs. Find a schedule that works for you and stick to it like peanut butter to jelly.

STAYING MOTIVATED AND ACCOUNTABLE

Staying motivated can be challenging, especially when arthritis pain flares up. But don't give up! Keep your eye on the prize and remind yourself of the benefits of exercise for your arthritis. Stay accountable by setting specific, measurable goals and enlisting a workout buddy, family member, or professional to support and encourage you along the way.

EVALUATING PROGRESS AND ADJUSTING YOUR PLAN AS NEEDED

Periodically evaluate your progress as you continue on your arthritis management. Be honest with yourself about how well you're sticking to your exercise plan and whether you're experiencing improvements in pain or joint function. If you're not seeing the results you'd hoped for, don't be afraid to adjust your plan. Remember, you are setting "milestones," not "marathon stones." Though this is a long race, set a pace you can manage and make any changes you need. Just keep striving for the goal.

FROM COUCH POTATO TO ARTHRITIS EXERCISE AFICIONADO

Managing arthritis can feel like a never-ending battle, but with the right approach to exercise, you can become the hero of your arthritis story. In this section, we'll guide you through incorporating arthritis-friendly exercises into your workouts and tracking your progress and pain levels. So, lace up your sneakers and let's tackle arthritis one workout at a time!

ARTHRITIS-FRIENDLY EXERCISES FOR YOUR WORKOUTS

Incorporating arthritis-friendly exercises into your workouts is essential for maintaining an active lifestyle while managing arthritis symptoms. Keep in mind the recommendations we discussed earlier: focus on aerobic exercises, strengthening exercises, and flexibility and balance exercises. For an extra dose of motivation, consider joining a group class or enlisting a workout buddy. Not only will you have fun exercising together, but you'll also have someone to empathize with over sore muscles and stiff joints.

MONITORING PROGRESS AND PAIN LEVELS OVER TIME

As your arthritis exercise starts, it's crucial to monitor your progress and pain levels. Keep a journal or use a fitness app to record your workouts, noting any changes in your arthritis symptoms. Are your pain levels decreasing? Is your range of motion improving? Can you do more reps or walk longer distances? These insights will help you fine-tune your exercise routine and stay motivated to keep going. After all, there's nothing more satisfying than witnessing the fruits of your labor.

Some arthritis-friendly exercises to consider incorporating into your routine include:

1. *Water aerobics or swimming*: These low-impact activities provide excellent aerobic exercise while minimizing stress on your joints.
2. *Gentle yoga or tai chi*: Both practices promote flexibility, balance, and relaxation, making them ideal for those with arthritis.
3. *Resistance band exercises*: Strengthening your muscles with resistance bands can help support your joints and reduce arthritis symptoms.
4. *Seated leg lifts or seated marches*: These exercises help strengthen the muscles around the hips and knees, providing support for joints affected by arthritis.
5. *Walking*: A simple, low-impact activity that improves cardiovascular health and strengthens muscles without putting excessive strain on your joints.

As always, consult your doctor or physical therapist before starting a new exercise routine, especially if you have arthritis or other health concerns. They can provide recommendations for exercises that are safe and effective for your specific situation. And remember, it's essential to listen to your body and adjust as needed to ensure a positive and beneficial exercise experience.

KEY TAKEAWAYS

1. Exercise is a powerful tool in managing arthritis, helping to alleviate pain and improve joint function.
2. Incorporating a balanced mix of aerobic, strengthening, and flexibility exercises into your routine is essential for arthritis management.
3. Listening to your body and working with a professional can help you create a safe and effective exercise plan tailored to your needs.
4. Staying consistent and committed to your arthritis exercise routine is crucial for long-term success and improved quality of life.
5. Tracking your progress and pain levels can provide valuable insights and motivation to keep you pushing forward with your exercise routine.

FINAL THOUGHTS

I know the pain that stiffness and inflammation can deliver. In the past, I have taken my fair share of Nonsteroidal Anti-Inflammatory Drugs (NSAIDs) – you know the ones I speak of – and occasionally I still take a couple after an especially physical day. But, over time they can do more damage to your body than the relief they deliver. Arthritis may appear to be an insurmountable obstacle, but you possess the power to take control and enhance your quality of life. Embrace the advantages of exercise and make a commitment to prioritize your health. Bear in mind that you are not alone on this excursion, and with the proper mindset and approach, you can overcome the challenges posed by arthritis and reclaim your vitality. So, lace up those sneakers, unroll your yoga mat, and immerse yourself in your new, arthritis-friendly exercise routine. Your joints will undoubtedly be grateful!

Arthritis is only one of the many types of pain that can be alleviated through exercise. In our next chapter, we'll examine into how exercise can also be a game-changer in managing pain from different sources as well as chronic pain. Prepare to uncover even more reasons to make exercise an enduring aspect of your life.

9

THE LANGUAGE OF PAIN: FROM ACUTE TO CHRONIC – PAIN HAS MANY FACES

P ain: It's one of the many four-letter words that summarize a vast collection of our own human experience. Pain is routinely perceived as an unwelcome visitor, an intruder that interrupts our lives and leaves us searching, sometimes begging for relief. It's kind of like that nosy second cousin, or neighbor who appears unannounced about the time we sit down to watch a ball game and wants to talk about some innocuous subject and can't take a subtle hint to leave. But what is pain, really? How can we understand it in order to live with it, conquer it, or engage in activities that help us cope?

At its core, pain is a protective mechanism. It is our body's way of communicating that something is wrong, whether an illness, injury, or other bodily aggravation. As pain signals travel through our nervous system, warning us to potential harm, it quietly and gently encourages us to seek some sort of intervention. Right? The pain I speak of screams at us and incites a potential riot if action is not immediately taken. Sometimes it just lingers. We all have our own special region that dominates the pain conversation. No matter, this crucial function is what has allowed humans to survive and advance; it teaches us to avoid hazards and prioritize self-preservation. [Remember Dopamine? How it's always seeking pleasure, while our bodies are tied up with our brains and they can't decide who's in charge, the body, or the brain?]

Not all pain is created equal. Acute pain, for instance, is a sudden, sharp sensation that typically lessens once the underlying issue is resolved. Chronic pain, on the other hand, lingers long past its expected expiration date, staying for months or even years. The latter can be particularly challenging to manage, as it often escapes a clear-cut cause or practical remedy.

So, how can we navigate the complex landscape of pain? I believe first step is to understand that pain is an inherently subjective experience. What may feel like a dull ache to one person could be a searing, unbearable agony to another. Recognizing that each individual's pain is valid and distinctive, we must approach its management with a personalized, multi-layered approach.

Living with pain is at best, an exercise in resilience. It asks us to acknowledge its presence (never a problem for me) and accepting that it may never entirely disappear. This acceptance, though challenging, enables us to focus on what we can control, and that is our response to pain. With a proactive approach of exercise, relaxation, and maintaining a healthy lifestyle, we can foster a sense of control in our pursuit of easing pain.

Conquering pain, on the other hand, involves actively pursuing interventions that alleviate or lessen our discomfort. This might involve working with healthcare professionals to explore medication, physical therapy, or alternative treatments like acupuncture. If you have gotten this far into this book you may have realized that it is my intent to push you to that uncomfortable zone where you're on the edge of either using it as a door stop or following through with the concepts I've presented. It is in that moment of time when you decide if this is all a load of BS, or I need to start taking better care of myself. You've got to stay open to different options and be determined in your pursuit of not only relief from pain, but also better health.

Lastly, engaging in activities that help us cope with pain can be transformative. Creative outlets like art, writing, or music can serve as powerful mediums for expressing our experiences and connecting with others who share our battles.

Let's face it, pain is a complex and multifaceted sensation that demands an individual approach. But understanding its nature, recognizing its subjectivity, and exploring different strategies for living with it, conquering it, or coping through supportive activities, we can promote a sense of liberation and resilience. Pain may be an inevitable part of the human experience, but it doesn't need to define us. Instead, it can serve as a catalyst for growth, self-discovery, and connection with others who walk similar paths.

TRIUMPHING OVER PERSISTENT PAIN

As you stride into the milestone of fifty years, (that's half a century you know), you've had a front row seat in life's abundant challenges – a majority of them, to be sure. From stretched muscles and twisted ankles to shattered bones, dislocations, stitches, and everything else that lies between, you've likely weathered your fair share of injuries. Some of these misfortunes can leave behind a lasting truckload of pain if not addressed.

Thankfully, by incorporating specific exercises into your routine, you can be enabled to target those troublesome spots and manage the ache they produce. I want to explore how physical activity can become your new secret weapon.

In this segment, I will shed light on the root causes of chronic pain and inflammation and outline how tailored exercise allows you to tackle these issues head-on with confidence.

UNDERSTANDING CHRONIC PAIN

Chronic pain is an unpleasant sensation that lasts for at least twelve weeks, often persisting beyond the normal healing time of an injury. If you thought you were the only one suffering, think again! According to the Centers for Disease Control and Prevention (CDC), about twenty percent of adults in the United States have chronic pain, while eight percent experience high-impact chronic pain that limits their daily activities (CDC, 2018).

So, what causes this persistent pain? There are many culprits, including:

1. *Injuries:* Old injuries that didn't heal properly can lead to chronic pain. A classic example is whiplash, which can cause ongoing neck pain if not treated correctly.
2. *Arthritis:* This inflammation of the joints can cause chronic pain in various parts of the body, such as the hands, knees, and hips.

3. *Fibromyalgia:* This condition causes widespread muscle pain and tenderness, often accompanied by fatigue and sleep disturbances.
4. *Nerve damage:* Conditions like diabetes or injuries can damage nerves, leading to chronic pain. One common type is diabetic neuropathy, which affects the nerves in the legs and feet.
5. *Migraines:* These severe headaches can cause chronic pain in some individuals, lasting for hours or even days.
6. *Cancer:* Tumors can press on nerves or other structures, causing pain. In some cases, treatments like chemotherapy or radiation therapy can also contribute to chronic pain.

THE INFLAMMATION FACTOR IN PERSISTENT PAIN

Inflammation takes center stage in this continuous drama. It's your body's instinctive reaction to injuries or infections, helping protect and heal the affected region. But when inflammation runs amok, it can actually intensify pain, creating a relentless loop.

Inflammation sets off the release of chemicals known as "cytokines." These substances heighten nerve sensitivity and make it easier for pain signals to travel. In some instances, inflammation can even result in adhesions – bands of scar tissue that limit movement and bring about discomfort.

Before we examine the realm of exercise as a strategy for easing pain, it's vital to recognize that everyone's experience with pain is distinct. If you're grappling with chronic pain, it's essential to consult a medical expert – a doctor or physical therapist – who can evaluate your specific circumstances and suggest the most suitable plan of action. They can advise you on the appropriate exercises to undertake, along with the correct form and technique to employ, which will help you steer clear of additional injuries and attain the most favorable outcomes.

HOW EXERCISE HELPS CHRONIC PAIN

You might be thinking, "Exercise? With chronic pain? Are you nuts?" But bear with me! Exercise is not only beneficial for overall health, but it can also be a powerful tool in your battle against pain and chronic pain specifically. Here's how:

1. *Strengthens muscles:* Exercise helps to build and maintain muscle strength, which can provide better support for your joints and reduce the strain on painful areas.
2. *Increases flexibility:* Stretching and flexibility exercises can improve your range of motion, making it easier to move and reducing pain.
3. *Improves circulation:* Regular exercise boosts blood flow, which can help to deliver oxygen and nutrients to your muscles and joints, promoting healing and reducing pain.
4. *Releases endorphins:* Physical activity triggers the release of endorphins – the body's natural painkillers – which can help to block pain signals and boost your mood.
5. *Promotes better sleep:* Exercise can improve sleep quality, which is crucial for pain management and overall well-being.

THE SCIENCE BEHIND EXERCISE AND PAIN RELIEF

The relationship between exercise and pain relief is more than just anecdotal. Research has shown that regular exercise can help to reduce chronic pain in several ways (Geneen et al., 2017).

For instance, studies have found that exercise can decrease inflammation, which, as we mentioned earlier, plays a significant role in chronic pain. Exercise also helps to increase pain tolerance by altering pain perception in the brain [thank you, Dopamine]. In short, exercise can change how your brain processes pain signals, making it less sensitive to pain (Walker, 2023).

TYPES OF EXERCISES SUITABLE FOR LINGERING PAIN RELIEF

When it comes to exercising with chronic pain, not all workouts are created equal. Some exercises may be more suitable for your specific pain condition than others. Generally, low-impact activities are recommended for chronic pain sufferers, as they are gentler on the joints and muscles. Some examples include:

1. *Aerobic exercises:* Low-impact aerobic exercises, such as walking, swimming, or cycling, can help to improve overall fitness and reduce pain.
2. *Strength training:* Using light weights or resistance bands to build muscle strength can provide better support for your joints and reduce the strain on painful areas.

3. *Flexibility exercises:* Stretching and yoga can improve your range of motion, making it easier to move and reducing pain.
4. *Balance exercises:* Improving balance can help to prevent falls and reduce the risk of further injury.

EXERCISES FOR CONSTANT PAIN – SOME RELIEF

Depending on your specific pain condition, certain exercises may be more beneficial than others. Here are some examples of targeted exercises for common types of chronic pain at the end of this chapter.

1. *Back pain:* Gentle stretches, core strengthening exercises, and low-impact aerobics activities can help to alleviate back pain.
2. *Arthritis:* Range-of-motion exercises, strength training, and low-impact aerobics activities can help to reduce joint pain and stiffness.
3. *Fibromyalgia:* A combination of low-impact aerobic exercises, strength training, and stretching can help to manage widespread pain and fatigue.
4. *Neuropathy:* Balance exercises, along with low-impact aerobics activities, can help to improve nerve function and reduce pain.

To choose the most effective exercise for your specific pain condition, consult with a medical professional or physical therapist. They can assess your individual situation and recommend suitable exercises based on your needs, abilities, and goals.

When exercising with chronic pain, safety should be your

top priority. Here are some precautions and safety measures to keep in mind:

1. *Start slow:* Gradually increase the intensity and duration of your workouts to avoid over exertion and prevent further injury.
2. *Listen to your body:* Pay attention to how your body feels during and after exercise. If you experience increased pain or discomfort, it might be a sign that you're pushing too hard or performing an unsuitable exercise. It also may take some time to get your body used to that exercise, push to the edge, but don't go over it.
3. *Warm-up and cool-down:* Always warm-up before exercising to prepare your muscles and joints for physical activity. Similarly, cool down afterward to help your body recover and prevent muscle soreness.
4. *Use proper form and technique:* Incorrect form can lead to further injury or exacerbate existing pain. Work with a physical therapist or qualified fitness professional to ensure you're performing exercises correctly.
5. *Modify exercises as needed:* Some exercises may need to be adapted to accommodate your specific pain condition or limitations. A physical therapist or fitness professional can help you make the necessary modifications.
6. *Stay consistent:* Consistency is key when it comes to managing chronic pain through exercise. Stick to a regular exercise routine and be patient – it may take time to see improvements in your pain levels.

While it may seem counterintuitive, exercise can be a powerful ally in your fight against chronic pain. By understanding the root causes of your pain and incorporating targeted exercises into your routine, you can work toward improved pain management and overall well-being. Just remember to consult with a medical professional [not YouTube] before starting any new exercise routine, and always prioritize safety when working out.

TIPS AND TRICKS FOR EXERCISING WITH PERSISTENT PAIN

When you're dealing with ongoing pain, jumping headfirst into a rigorous exercise routine is not a good idea. Pain is a great motivator; it can also hinder any desire to make your body do things that merely perpetuate the crummy feeling. Begin with low-impact exercises like walking, swimming, or gentle yoga, and gradually increase the intensity and duration of your workouts as your pain levels improve and your body adapts. (Note on gentle Yoga: I first tried Yoga while on a cruise, I was the only man in the "sanctuary." "Simple stretching and easy poses," they said. Half an hour and it kicked my butt! So, start slow and avoid the humiliation I endured. I was sweatin' like a racehorse after the Kentucky Derby.)

Using proper form and technique during exercise is crucial for preventing further injury and ensuring pain relief. Poor form can strain your muscles and joints, potentially aggravating your pain. To be sure you're exercising correctly, consider working with a physical therapist or a qualified fitness professional who can guide you through the proper techniques and help you avoid common mistakes.

One of the most important aspects of exercising with chronic pain is learning to listen to your body. Be open to adjusting your workout routine as needed and remember that it's okay to take breaks or decrease the intensity if you're experiencing too much discomfort.

Managing chronic pain through exercise requires consistency and patience. Stick to a regular exercise routine and be prepared for the fact that it may take time to see improvements in your pain levels. Celebrate small victories, like completing a workout without worsening your pain or noticing slight improvements in your pain levels and stay patient with the process.

CREATING A PERSONALIZED EXERCISE PLAN FOR PERSISTENT PAIN RELIEF

The first step in creating a personalized exercise plan for chronic pain relief is to identify the root cause of your pain. Was it caused by an injury, illness, or another underlying issue? Understanding the cause of your pain will help you and your healthcare provider determine the most appropriate exercises and strategies for managing your pain.

Once you've received clearance from your healthcare provider, start incorporating targeted exercises into your routine. These exercises should be chosen based on their ability to address the underlying cause of your pain and promote healing. For example, if you're dealing with lower back pain, you might include exercises that strengthen your core muscles and improve your flexibility and hip mobility.

As you embark on your personalized exercise plan, it's essential to track your progress and pain levels over time. Keep a journal or use a smartphone app to record your workouts, pain levels, and any changes in your symptoms. This information will be invaluable in helping you and your healthcare team fine-tune your exercise plan and gauge the effectiveness of your efforts.

Exercising with chronic pain might seem daunting, but with the right approach and guidance, it can be a powerful tool for managing pain and improving your quality of life.

KEY TAKEAWAYS

1. Pain is a complex issue, but exercise can be a powerful tool in managing it and improving your quality of life.
2. Starting slow and progressing gradually, as well as using proper form and technique, is crucial for exercising safely with chronic pain.
3. Listening to your body and being open to adjusting your workout routine as needed is essential for finding what works best for your specific pain condition.
4. Consistency and patience are key when using exercise to manage pain, as improvement takes time to become noticeable.
5. Creating a personalized exercise plan and working closely with your healthcare team can help you take control of chronic pain and work toward a healthier and happier future.

FINAL THOUGHTS

The passage to overcoming pain through exercise may seem challenging but remember that you're not alone. By taking small, consistent steps and working closely with your health-care team, you can make a significant, positive change in your life. Embrace the power of exercise and be patient with yourself as you navigate this path. With determination, perseverance, and the right approach, you can conquer chronic pain and unlock a new level of well-being.

It's important to note that treatment recommendations should be based on your individual specific condition and medical history, so always talk to a healthcare professional for personalized advice.

Exercise can be extremely beneficial for managing different types of chronic pain, it helps to improve strength, flexibility, and overall well-being. I have listed five types of chronic pain conditions that can be positively impacted by exercise and a recommended exercise for each:

1. *Osteoarthritis:*

- Low-impact aerobic exercises, like walking or swimming
- Strength training exercises targeting the affected joints
- Flexibility and range of motion exercises, like yoga or tai chi

2. Fibromyalgia:

- Low-impact aerobic exercises, such as walking, swimming, or cycling
- Gentle strength training exercises, like resistance bands or light weights
- Stretching and relaxation exercises, like yoga or Pilates

3. Chronic lower back pain:

- Core-strengthening exercises, like planks and bridges
- Low-impact aerobic exercises, such as walking or swimming
- Flexibility and stretching exercises, like hamstring stretches or cat-cow poses

4. Chronic neck pain:

- Gentle range of motion exercises for the neck
- Isometric exercises, like pressing the head against resistance
- Strengthening exercises for the upper back and shoulders, like seated rows or shoulder shrugs

5. Diabetic peripheral neuropathy:

- Low-impact aerobic exercises, such as walking, swimming, or cycling
- Balance exercises, like standing on one foot or using a balance board

- Gentle strength training exercises, like resistance bands or light weights

As always, before starting any exercise program, it's essential to consult with a healthcare professional or a physical therapist to ensure that the chosen exercises are safe and appropriate for your specific condition. They can help design an individualized exercise program tailored to your needs and monitor your progress. Remember to start slow and gradually increase the intensity and duration of your exercises to avoid injury or aggravating your pain.

The following is some general information on pain descriptors and potential treatments for inflammation-related pain. Remember to consult a healthcare professional for advice tailored to your specific situation.

1. *Throbbing pain*: This pain is often described as a pulsing sensation. Over-the-counter anti-inflammatory medications like ibuprofen may help reduce swelling and pain.
2. *Aching pain*: A dull, continuous pain that can be managed with hot or cold therapy, physical therapy, or pain-relief medications.
3. *Sharp pain*: Sudden, intense pain that may be alleviated with rest, ice, compression, and elevation (RICE) or prescription pain medications if necessary.
4. *Stabbing pain*: Intense pain that can be treated similarly to sharp pain, with RICE, pain-relief medications, or anti-inflammatory drugs.

5. *Burning pain:* Pain that feels like a hot sensation. Topical analgesics like lidocaine or capsaicin cream may offer relief.
6. *Tingling or pins-and-needles pain*: This may indicate nerve involvement. Treatment can include nerve pain medications like gabapentin, physical therapy, or acupuncture.
7. *Electric shock-like pain:* Sudden, intense pain that may respond to nerve pain medications, TENS (transcutaneous electrical nerve stimulation) therapy, or relaxation techniques.
8. *Shooting pain:* Pain that travels along a nerve pathway, which may be managed with nerve pain medications, stretching, or acupuncture.
9. *Radiating pain*: Pain that spreads from the source. Treatment options include anti-inflammatory medications, physical therapy, or targeted injections.
10. *Cramping pain:* Involuntary muscle contractions that may be alleviated with massage, heat therapy, or muscle relaxants.
11. *Stiffness-related pain:* Pain resulting from reduced mobility. Gentle stretching, heat therapy, and anti-inflammatory medications can help.
12. *Swelling-related pain:* Discomfort caused by inflammation. NSAIDs (nonsteroidal anti-inflammatory drugs), ice therapy, and compression may provide relief.
13. *Tender pain:* Pain experienced upon touch or pressure. Treatment may involve rest, RICE, or gentle stretching.

14. *Sore pain:* A dull, achy pain that can be managed with heat therapy, massage, or over-the-counter pain medications.
15. *Heavy or deep pain:* A feeling of weight or pressure, which may be alleviated with massage, heat therapy, or pain-relief medications.

I think I've beat this topic into submission and have explored the benefits of exercise for managing different types of pain. Next, I want to examine another crucial aspect of maintaining a healthy lifestyle – SLEEP. In the next chapter, we'll consider how incredibly important quality sleep is for overall health and well-being and provide practical tips for improving your sleep habits.

10

THE POWER OF SLEEP – YOUR SECRET WEAPON FOR A HEALTHIER LIFE

S*leep* – that glorious, elusive, and often undervalued wonder. It's the comforting embrace we all yearn for after an exhausting day, yet somehow, it perpetually seems to slip through our fingers. In this chapter, I will examine the puzzling realm of sleep, demystify its complexities, and reveal its crucial role in maintaining our overall health and wellbeing, both physical and mental.

THE SCIENCE OF SLEEP: UNCOVERING ITS SIGNIFICANCE

We've all come across the adage, "You snooze, you lose." Surprisingly, the reality is quite the contrary – "You snooze, you triumph." Why, you ask? It's because sleep is one of the most essential components in life for preserving both our physical and mental health. Envision it as your body's personal superhero, arriving just in time to rescue your system by repairing and refreshing it.

So, what occurs as we drift off into the world of dreams? Well, sleep consists of a couple of stages, each with its own distinct purpose. The two primary types of sleep are rapid eye movement (REM) sleep and non-rapid eye movement (NREM) sleep, which can be further split into three phases (Cherry & Blackmer, n.d.). During NREM sleep, our bodies concentrate on physical renewal, while REM sleep is concerned with mental and emotional repair. I know, it's as though we need our brains and emotions sent to the shop for service. In essence, sleep is akin to an all-inclusive spa experience for your body and mind.

Given the extraordinary benefits of sleep, why do we regularly treat it as an annoying guest we can't wait to evict? Part of the answer lies in the hectic nature of modern life. With the whirlwind of work, socializing, and binge-watching our favorite shows (I'm guilty too!), sleep is often demoted and pushed to the background. As a young man I had a bad case of FOMO, fear of missing out. I wanted to experience as much life as I could cram into my youth. And cram I did, not unlike you. Regrettably, neglecting our sleep comes with a substantial cost, and it involves more than having to retake that stupid geometry class in college. The consequences of being sleep deficient are far from trivial. It results in impaired cognitive function, mood fluctuations, weakened immune systems, and a heightened risk of chronic health issues such as obesity, diabetes, and heart disease. In short, skimping on sleep is akin to poking a bear with a stick – you're inviting trouble.

In the subsequent sections, I will examine the advantages of adequate sleep, common sleep challenges and their remedies, and how to design a personalized sleep strategy to ensure you're seizing those invaluable moments of slumber like a seasoned expert.

THE BENEFITS OF GETTING ENOUGH SLEEP

The sensation of waking up after a truly restful night's sleep is sweet. You feel refreshed, rejuvenated, and ready to tackle whatever the day throws your way. But did you know that sleep is more than just a luxury or an escape from our daily grind? It's a powerhouse that provides numerous benefits, both for our mental and physical health. In this section, we'll dive deep into the myriad of advantages that come with getting enough sleep, from boosting our memory to supporting our immune system. So, fluff up those pillows and get cozy because we're about to explore the marvelous world of sleep benefits.

Improved Memory and Cognitive Performance

If you've ever pulled an all-nighter, you know how difficult it is to concentrate and remember things the next day. That's because sleep is essential for the consolidation of memories and learning. During slumber, your brain processes and organizes the information you've acquired throughout the day, making it easier to recall later on. So, if you want to ace that trivia night or remember where you put your car keys, make sure you're getting enough sleep!

Enhanced Immune System Function

While you snooze, your body is hard at work repairing and regenerating cells, including those responsible for your immune system. Adequate sleep has been linked to a stronger immune response, which can help you fight off infections and keep you healthy. So, the next time someone tells you to "sleep it off," they might be on to something!

Better Mood and Emotional Regulation

We've all experienced the grumpiness that comes with a restless night, but did you know that chronic sleep deprivation can lead to more severe mood disturbances, like anxiety and depression? On the flip side, getting enough rest can improve your emotional stability and even make you more resilient to stress. So, if you want to keep your cool when life throws you curveballs, be sure to prioritize your beauty sleep.

Increased Energy Levels and Physical Performance

It's no secret that a good night's rest can leave you feeling energized and ready to tackle the day. In fact, sleep is crucial for muscle recovery and athletic performance. Whether you're training for a marathon or just trying to keep up with your grandkids, getting enough sleep will help you stay in tip-top shape.

COMMON SLEEP PROBLEMS AND SOLUTIONS

Sleep disorders, such as insomnia, sleep apnea, and restless legs syndrome, can wreak havoc on your sleep quality and overall well-being. If you're struggling to fall asleep, stay asleep, or wake up feeling refreshed, it's essential to consult a healthcare professional for a proper diagnosis and treatment plan (Sleep Foundation, n.d.).

Several factors can influence how well you sleep, including your bedtime routine, sleep environment, and even the foods you eat. To set yourself up for a restful night, pay attention to your habits and adjust as needed (Mayo Clinic, n.d.).

TIPS FOR IMPROVING SLEEP HYGIENE AND CREATING AN OPTIMAL SLEEP ENVIRONMENT

Practicing good sleep hygiene can help you fall asleep faster and stay asleep longer. Some tips for creating a sleep-friendly environment include but are not limited to:

- Maintaining a consistent sleep schedule
- Keeping your bedroom cool, dark, and quiet
- Avoiding caffeine and alcohol close to bedtime
- Establishing a relaxing pre-sleep routine

If racing thoughts (monkey brain) or stress are keeping you awake at night, consider incorporating relaxation techniques, like deep breathing exercises, progressive muscle relaxation, or meditation, into your bedtime routine. Managing stress during the day can also help you sleep more soundly at night, so don't hesitate to seek out stress-reduction strategies that work for you. There are a wide variety of "supplements" that are advertised as being "the remedy" for sleepless nights. We all know how advertising works. Identify the optimal solution that aligns with your specific needs and objectives, and then persistently stick to it.

DETERMINING THE RIGHT AMOUNT OF SLEEP FOR YOU

It turns out that sleep needs change as we age. As much as we'd like to believe we can still get by on the four hours of sleep we survived on in college, our aging bodies beg to differ. The National Sleep Foundation has done us all a solid by providing age-specific sleep recommendations:

- Newborns (0-3 months): 14-17 hours
- Infants (4-11 months): 12-15 hours
- Toddlers (1-2 years): 11-14 hours
- Preschoolers (3-5 years): 10-13 hours
- School-age children (6-13 years): 9-11 hours
- Teenagers (14-17 years): 8-10 hours
- Young adults (18-25 years): 7-9 hours
- Adults (26-64 years): 7-9 hours
- Older adults (65+ years): 7-8 hours

Don't take these numbers as gospel; they're merely guidelines. You've probably noticed that some people can function just fine on five or six hours of sleep, while others need a full nine hours to avoid resembling a caffeine-addicted zombie. That's because individual differences, such as genetics, lifestyle, and health conditions, can impact how much sleep a person needs.

For instance, some lucky folks have a genetic mutation that allows them to function on less sleep than others. Talk about winning the genetic lottery! On the flip side, someone with a sleep disorder or chronic health condition may require more sleep to feel truly rested.

Start by paying attention to your body. If you're constantly feeling tired and relying on caffeine to get through the day, you might need to latch on to a few more Z's each night.

Here are some tips for adjusting your sleep schedule:

- Establish a consistent bedtime and wake-up time, even on weekends. This will help regulate your body's internal clock, making it easier to fall asleep and wake up feeling refreshed.
- Create a relaxing bedtime routine to signal to your body that it's time to wind down. This might include reading a book, taking a warm bath, or practicing gentle stretches.
- Make your sleep environment as comfortable as possible by investing in a supportive mattress, cozy bedding, and blackout curtains to keep your room dark.

TRACKING AND IMPROVING YOUR SLEEP

You've probably heard that magical number before: eight hours of sleep per night. But let's be honest, not everyone fits into that neat little box. In fact, the amount of sleep we need can vary greatly depending on factors like age, lifestyle, and individual differences. So, how can you determine the right amount of sleep for you? In this section, we've provided you with age-specific sleep recommendations. Now let's delve into the factors that could influence your unique sleep requirements. Moreover, we'll equip you with strategies to adjust your sleep schedule to meet your individual needs. It's time to unlock the secret to your perfect night's sleep!

Assessing Your Current Sleep Satisfaction Levels

Before you can start improving your sleep, it's important to evaluate your current sleep satisfaction levels. For two weeks, keep a sleep journal to record how well-rested you feel each morning, as well as any factors that may have influenced your sleep quality (e.g., stress, caffeine, alcohol, or a noisy environment).

Incorporating Sleep Improvement Tips Into Your Nightly Routine

After evaluating your sleep satisfaction levels, it's time to put some of the tips mentioned earlier into action. Choose two or more strategies to improve your sleep, such as establishing a consistent sleep schedule or creating a relaxing bedtime routine. Stick to these changes for at least two weeks to give your body time to adjust.

Tracking the Changes in Your Sleep Satisfaction Levels Over Time

While you implement your sleep improvement strategies, continue to track your sleep satisfaction levels in your sleep diary. This will allow you to monitor your progress and see whether your changes are making a difference.

Adjusting Your Sleep Improvement Strategies Based On the Results

After two weeks of implementing your sleep improvement strategies, assess whether your sleep satisfaction levels have improved. If you're still struggling to get the rest you need, consider trying different strategies or seeking professional help from a sleep specialist.

Remember, sleep is a highly individualized process, and what works for one person may not work for another. Be patient and keep experimenting until you find the approach that works best for you

KEY TAKEAWAYS

1. Sleep plays a vital role in maintaining our physical and mental health, and it's essential to prioritize it in our daily lives.
2. Getting enough sleep has numerous benefits, including improved memory, enhanced immune function, better mood, and increased energy levels.
3. Common sleep problems can be addressed through proper sleep hygiene, creating an optimal sleep environment, and managing stress.
4. Determining the right amount of sleep for your unique needs involves considering age-specific recommendations and individual differences.
5. Tracking and improving your sleep can be achieved by incorporating sleep improvement tips into your routine, monitoring sleep satisfaction levels, and adjusting as needed.

FINAL THOUGHTS

Sleep is an often-underestimated aspect of a healthy lifestyle, but it holds immense power in shaping our well-being. As you continue to age gracefully, remember to give your body and mind the rest they deserve. Consult with your healthcare provider about taking any supplement as it can interact with other medications. With the knowledge you've gained in this chapter, you're now equipped to make lasting, positive changes to your sleep habits.

In the next chapter, we'll confront some of the fears that come with aging and explore strategies to navigate this phase of life with confidence and resilience. Sleep well.

11

THE SILENT KILLER LURKING WITHIN

P icture this: you're settled in the heart of a family gathering, savoring the pleasant flavors of a homemade meal, and enjoying the gentle hum of friendly banter. The conversation takes a turn and lands on the subject of your friend's recurring health issues. As you disclose that he's currently in the hospital, an unexpected hush descends upon the room. The reason? A stealthy adversary that inhabits each of us, a concealed danger biding its time to strike – high blood pressure. As we grow older, regulating our blood pressure becomes increasingly difficult, and the risks escalate. Don't dial 911 yet. A fusion of physical activity and a healthful diet can aid us in subjugating this foe, ensuring our vigor and vitality as we sail through our golden years.

In this chapter, I will examine the terrain of high blood pressure, investigating its nature, the significance of its management, and how you can seize control of this naughty little dude before it asserts dominance over you.

DECODING HIGH BLOOD PRESSURE

When you've had your blood pressure measured, you might have encountered a pair of numbers, such as "120 over 80" or something similar. The initial figure represents your systolic pressure, measuring the pressure in your arteries when your heart contracts. The latter number corresponds to your diastolic pressure, assessing the pressure in your arteries during the heart's relaxation phase between beats. So, what factors contribute to these numbers climbing to unsafe altitudes?

High blood pressure, or hypertension, transpires when the force of blood against your artery walls remains consistently elevated. This can occur for a multitude of reasons, encompassing genetics, lifestyle choices, and even the natural aging process (CDC, n.d.).

I was at the dentist this week for my semi-annual clean and exam, the subject of this book came up. I was telling my hygienist what I was currently working on, and he told me they recently had a patient who was in for a surgical implant and needed anesthesia for the procedure. Of course, they take all their vitals prior to putting him under, his BP was 215/150, they took it again and the same result. They had to cancel the surgery. The patient said, and I quote, "But I feel fine." This is a very sneaky villain.

UNDERSTANDING HIGH BLOOD PRESSURE

To understand high blood pressure, we need to first understand how the arteries work. Arteries are like flexible pipes in your body that carry blood from your heart to the rest of your body. The blood pumped by your heart gives pressure to the artery walls similar to water being pushed through a garden hose. This pressure is important for blood to be able to reach all parts of your body and provide them with the oxygen and nutrients they need.

Now, imagine if your garden hose became narrower or if the water pump started pushing water with more force. The water pressure inside the hose would increase, right? The same thing happens in your body. High blood pressure, also known as hypertension, occurs when your heart has to pump harder, or the arteries become narrower, causing the blood to exert more pressure on the artery walls. The muscular layer in the arterial walls contracts and relaxes to regulate blood flow and pressure. Contraction of the arteries (vasoconstriction) narrows the blood vessels, increasing blood pressure, while relaxation (vasodilation) widens the blood vessels, reducing blood pressure.

There are a few symptoms of high blood pressure, but the tricky part is, most people won't experience any. That's why high blood pressure is often called the "silent killer," because it quietly damages your body before obvious symptoms develop. However, in some cases, symptoms can include severe headaches, fatigue, irregular heartbeat, chest pain, difficulty breathing, or blood in the urine.

As for remedies, there are several options for lowering blood pressure:

1. *Lifestyle Changes*: This is the first and most important step. It involves eating a healthy diet (particularly a low salt one), regular exercise, maintaining a healthy weight, limiting alcohol, reducing stress, and avoiding tobacco.

2. *Medications*: If lifestyle changes aren't enough, there are various medications available, such as diuretics, ACE inhibitors, and calcium channel blockers. The specific drug or combination of drugs depends on the patient's overall health, the presence of any other diseases, and the specific characteristics of their high blood pressure.

3. *Regular Monitoring*: Regular check-ups with your healthcare provider is key to manage high blood pressure. They'll monitor your blood pressure regularly and adjust your treatment plan if necessary.

Remember, each of us is different. What works best will depend on a person's specific health situation, so any changes should be made under the guidance of a healthcare provider.

Finally, it's also important to know that our age, family history, and race can increase the risk of high blood pressure. It's not always about your lifestyle – sometimes, it's just the cards we've been dealt. But by taking care of your health and working closely with your doctor, high blood pressure can often be effectively managed.

THE ROLE OF MAGNESIUM IN BLOOD PRESSURE

Our arteries are not just simple tubes; they're actually quite dynamic and complex. Unlike our veins, they are made up of smooth muscle cells and elastic fibers that allow them to contract and expand as needed. This contraction and relaxation process helps to regulate blood pressure and distribute blood throughout the body.

When your heart beats, it pumps blood into the arteries,

causing them to expand. Then, in between heartbeats, the arteries contract to keep the blood moving. This is a continuous process. However, with high blood pressure, the arteries may have difficulty relaxing completely. This could be due to a variety of reasons, such as the buildup of plaque (a condition called atherosclerosis), or increased stiffness in the arteries due to aging. When the arteries can't relax completely, they become narrower, and the heart has to work harder to pump blood, which then leads to increased blood pressure.

Regarding magnesium, yes, it does play a significant role in the proper functioning of our bodies, including muscle function and the health of our arteries. Magnesium helps to regulate muscle contractions and relaxations by acting as a natural calcium blocker. In the context of arteries, this means it can help the smooth muscles in the artery walls relax, which can help to lower blood pressure (NIH, National Center of Biotechnology Information). I was put on magnesium to help manage my irregular heart rhythm; it has been added to my daily supplement routine. Further, several studies have suggested that a higher intake of magnesium may be associated with a lower risk of high blood pressure. However, it's important to note that while magnesium is beneficial, it's just one piece of the puzzle. A balanced diet, regular exercise, and a healthy lifestyle overall are crucial to maintaining healthy blood pressure levels.

As always, you should consult with your doctor before starting any new supplement regimen, including magnesium, because it can interact with certain medications and medical conditions.

THE HEALTH IMPLICATIONS AND RISKS LINKED TO HIGH BLOOD PRESSURE

You may be pondering, "What's the big deal about high blood pressure? Surely, my arteries can withstand a bit of pressure!" While that might hold some truth, but persistent high blood pressure can bring on numerous other health complications.

Initially, high blood pressure can inflict havoc on your blood vessels, rendering them less pliable and more susceptible to rupture or obstruction. Consequently, this may culminate in heart attacks, strokes, and renal failure. As if that isn't unnerving enough, hypertension can also trigger vision loss, sexual dysfunction, and memory issues (Mayo Clinic, 2021).

So, yeah it is kind of a big deal.

BLOOD PRESSURE CONTROL AND THE INFLUENCE OF AGE

As we advance in years, our blood vessels lose some suppleness, making it more challenging for our hearts to pump blood effectively. This can contribute to elevated blood pressure, rendering hypertension increasingly common among older individuals. In fact, the National Institute on Aging reveals that almost two-thirds of adults above the age of 60 suffer from high blood pressure. That's two out of three of every one of you reading this! Odds are, you have elevated BP. Get it checked, sooner than later.

But don't concede to a life of hypertension just yet; remember that age is merely a number. (Sorry for the clichés but sometimes they just work.) You possess the capability to take charge of your blood pressure and manage it effectively, even as you mature. All that's required is a hint of wisdom, a handful of sensible habits, and a bit of perseverance.

PREVENTING HIGH BLOOD PRESSURE

Have you ever come across the adage, "An ounce of prevention is worth a pound of cure"? This statement is particularly true for high blood pressure. In this segment, we'll probe into the enchanting realm of prevention, where well-balanced diets, consistent physical activity, and other lifestyle modifications serve as the cornerstone for holding off hypertension. So, strap in and prepare to uncover the secrets of sustaining healthy blood pressure levels and embracing your most fulfilling life.

THE SKILL OF EATING WELL FOR YOUR BLOOD PRESSURE

"You are what you eat" – another cliché, yes, but when it comes to blood pressure, its wisdom can't be brushed aside. An abundance of fruits, veggies, whole grains, and lean proteins can work wonders on those numbers. Enter the DASH diet (Dietary Approaches to Stop Hypertension) – a plan designed to help manage hypertension by embracing sea salt (adios to table salt with its impurities!) and upping your potassium and magnesium intake (NHLBI, n.d.).

A wholesome diet doesn't mean you must part ways with flavor. The world of blood pressure-friendly foods is vast and actually quite good. It's about making savvy choices – such as delicious and authentic whole grains. A bit of creativity and a tweak of enthusiasm will keep your taste buds happy while taming that pesky blood pressure.

*Quick word on table salt – even "ultra-pure NaCl" contains trace amounts of aluminum, arsenic, bromides, heavy metals, iron, magnesium, phosphates, and sulfates. So, yes, table salt isn't all that innocent.

I have compiled a partial list of foods that aid in maintaining a reasonable BP, and in some cases may even lower your numbers. There's a caveat to these foods and their role in resolving high blood pressure. I have friends who are in very good health, they eat well and exercise on a regular basis and still have some hypertension. Genetics, age, ethnicity, and overall health all play a role in your likelihood of developing high BP. If you are on any of the myriad of BP medications, please don't stop taking them just because you have changed your diet. Your doctor has prescribed them for a reason, so please, consult with them to form a strategy that can help ween you off those prescriptions. The best advice I have for you, and it's number one on the list, is to make a dietary changes that you can actually stick to so you can drop some weight. You should also begin an exercise routine. You can get healthy, but it's you who makes the decision.

1. Leafy greens (replacing iceberg lettuce):
2. Spinach
3. Kale (my wife made me put this in)
4. Swiss chard
5. Arugula
6. Romaine lettuce
7. Berries (replacing sugary snacks and processed fruit products):
8. Blueberries
9. Raspberries

10. Strawberries
11. Blackberries
12. Whole grains (replacing refined grains and white flour products):
13. Quinoa
14. Brown rice
15. Barley
16. Whole wheat
17. Oats (whole and rolled or steel cut)
18. Seeds and nuts (replacing unhealthy snacks and chips):
19. Almonds
20. Walnuts
21. Chia seeds
22. Pumpkin seeds
23. Fatty fish (replacing processed meats)
24. Salmon
25. Mackerel
26. Sardines
27. Tuna
28. Trout
29. Dairy (*in moderation*, we need some fats in our diet)
30. Whole milk
31. 4% milkfat yogurt
32. Real, not processed cheese
33. Cottage cheese
34. Olive oil (replacing unhealthy cooking seed oils and fats)
35. Extra virgin olive oil
36. Cold-pressed avocado oil

37. Seasonings (replacing table salt and sodium-laden condiments):
38. Fresh or dried herbs, such as basil, oregano, rosemary, and thyme
39. Spices, like turmeric, cumin, and paprika
40. Vinegar, such as apple cider vinegar or balsamic vinegar
41. Freshly ground black pepper
42. Sea salt

THE INFLUENCE OF REGULAR EXERCISE

All right let's face it – exercise might not be everyone's idea of fun. But when it comes to blood pressure, breaking a sweat can be a game-changer. Consistent physical activity strengthens your heart, making it more efficient at pumping blood. The good news is you don't have to spend an extensive amount of time at the gym to reap the benefits. If you start with brisk walks, swimming, or even dancing, they all can make a dip in your blood pressure. In the beginning, aim for a weekly period of 75 minutes of moderate aerobic workouts or 45 minutes of vigorous activity (resistance and/or weight training – I use kettlebells and resistance bands). Always remember, consistency is key. You can and should increase your time, weight, and reps as your endurance improves.

LIFESTYLE TWEAKS FOR A HEALTHIER YOU

Beyond diet and exercise, other lifestyle adjustments can help keep blood pressure at bay, i.e., stress management, ample sleep, and maybe putting the cork back in the bourbon bottle.

Don't overlook the power of social support! Rally friends and family who share your health-centered ambitions – it can make a world of difference. Enlist a workout buddy, find a support group, or share your crusade on social media. And remember, because you are now a dues paying, card carrying member of the "old guy club," we're all in this together.

KEEPING TABS ON BLOOD PRESSURE AS THE YEARS ROLL BY

We all like to think we're aging like fine wine. However, when it comes to blood pressure, the years can take a bit of a toll. If we want to age gracefully, it's essential to keep a vigilant eye on our blood pressure and adopt strategies to keep it in check. Lucky for you, I've got a handy assortment of tips and tricks up my sleeve to help you stay ahead in this game of life.

FREQUENT BLOOD PRESSURE CHECKS AND DECODING THE DIGITS

As we grow older, keeping tabs on our blood pressure becomes increasingly vital, and cracking the code behind those numbers is empowering (Mayo Clinic, n.d.). Generally, a healthy blood pressure hovers below 120/80 mm Hg. As I previously stated, the first figure, the systolic pressure, gauges the pressure in your arteries during heartbeats. The second one, the diastolic pressure, assesses the pressure in your arteries as your heart takes a break between beats.

Because the years are adding up, it's crucial to get your blood pressure checked at least semi-annually, or more often if you're prone to hypertension (American Heart Association, n.d.). You can get a BP cuff, they're pretty cheap, and take your own, just get trained on the correct technique and when to take it to get accurate readings. Remember, knowledge packs a punch. Being in the know about your digits can steer you toward well-informed choices concerning your health.

PHARMACEUTICALS AND THEIR PART IN TAMING BLOOD PRESSURE

I know popping pills isn't the highlight of your day but, occasionally, it's essential to keep your blood pressure within healthy limits. If lifestyle adjustments just aren't cutting the mustard, your doc might prescribe meds to help bring those numbers down.

There's a medley of medications out there, each working its magic in unique ways. Some ease up your blood vessels, while others decelerate your heart rate or trim down your body's fluid content. The crucial part is to collaborate with your healthcare professional to pinpoint the right medication and dosage tailored to your needs. And don't forget, consistency is vital, so don't skip those tablets.

That being said, the underlying motivation for this book is to get and then stay in good health. Taking different medications to ensure you are able to live life long and happy may be necessary, but my goal is to get you off them. Addressing the cause of your physical aliment with strategies that are effective and long-lasting, and not placing a Rx Band-Aid on the issue. Which, I'm sorry to say, is the standard these days in many physician-patient relationships. I have several good friends who are MD. They, too, want to see less of you in their office or on the operating table and more of you celebrating multiple more birthdays. However, they see people who have kind of "mailed it in." They've lost any hope of a healthy future. We are creatures of habit, some of those are slowly corroding our will to change our direction in life so we can have more of it. You want to change? Make it happen.

CRAFTING A TAILORED BLOOD PRESSURE MANAGEMENT STRATEGY

All righty then, it's time to get down to business and craft a custom-made blood pressure management plan that caters to your individual needs.

First things first, know your starting point. Get your blood pressure measured and take note of any risk factors in play, like a family history of hypertension, excess weight, or smoking habits. This intel will help you fine-tune your plan for maximum impact. (There is a section in your workbook/journal to record your BP.) Diet and exercise go hand in hand as your reliable allies in this blood pressure battle. Begin by infusing your meals with heart-friendly ingredients; I've listed some of them on a prior page. Oh, and keep an eye on table salt intake. When it comes to breaking a sweat, shoot for a minimum of 150 minutes (start with fewer minutes if necessary) of moderate-intensity aerobic exercise per week. This could be brisk walking, swimming, or dancing – pick your poison and hit the ground running!

It's vital to monitor your blood pressure as your management plan unfolds. Regular check-ins will help you gauge the progress you're making and pinpoint any aspects needing extra attention. Patience is a virtue – don't lose heart if your digits don't plummet overnight. Stay committed to your plan, and you'll be on the right path. It takes time to see results, but if you follow it, you will see results.

As you persistently assess your blood pressure, feel free to tweak your management strategy based on the outcomes. This could involve fine-tuning your food choices, switching up your exercise regimen, or discussing medication adjustments with your doc. Be adaptable and open to change in your approach.

And there you go! Equipped with a robust comprehension of high blood pressure and furnished with tactics for prevention and control, you're all set to seize control of your well-being and keep the silent killer at a safe distance. As you move on toward improved health and graceful aging, bear in mind that each tiny stride matters. Now, let's shift gears and look into another crucial component of maintaining our health as we age: safeguarding our hearts.

KEY TAKEAWAYS

1. High blood pressure is a silent and dangerous condition that can lead to severe health issues, particularly as you age.
2. Maintaining a healthy diet, exercising regularly, and adopting other lifestyle changes can help prevent and manage high blood pressure.
3. Understanding your blood pressure numbers and monitoring them regularly is crucial for staying in control of your health.
4. Knowing that positive lifestyle changes can lead to significant improvements in blood pressure control and overall health.

5. Developing a personalized blood pressure management plan and adapting it as needed is vital for maintaining good health as you age.

FINAL THOUGHTS

High blood pressure may be a silent killer, but you have the power to take charge of your health and protect yourself from its potentially devastating consequences. Remember, it's never too late to make a change. So, take control, adopt healthy habits, and start your trip toward better blood pressure management.

12

THE BLUEPRINT OF HEART HEALTH – PROTECTING THE CORE

I'm willing to bet when you were young and didn't have a firm grasp of the direction you wanted to go in life, some amateur philosophy major said, "Just follow your heart." You heard it enough that occasionally you followed that counsel and things didn't go well. Now, at this point in our life, we should actually prioritize safeguarding that tireless, beating engine at our core and follow its calling. It may need some much-deserved TLC. As we move on in life, there is a river, and it's swift, deep, and very wide. It is full of knowledge and information available to anyone who dares go near its ledge. If you've gotten this far into this book, it's time to jump, feet first and hold on to the lifeline and put into practice all that you've learned. Your life literally depends on your willingness to apply what you know. The Greeks have a word for it, *"sofia."* It means skilled intelligence, insight; the English is *"wisdom."*

In this chapter, we're going to dive into the realm of cholesterol and heart disease, illuminating the significance of grasping your cholesterol levels and how you can spring into action to keep your heart healthy and robust. So, let's place the power of prevention right into your hands (or should I say arteries)!

DECIPHERING CHOLESTEROL AND ITS INFLUENCE ON CARDIAC HEALTH

Cholesterol. Even the word can strike fear into the sturdiest of hearts, painting a picture of a health world's Darth Vader. But cholesterol isn't entirely the villain of the piece, as our bodies need cholesterol to function optimally. Cholesterol, a waxy, fat-like entity, is the secret behind the creation of hormones, vitamin D, and other substances vital for our bodies (Health-line, n.d.). So, why the notorious reputation? Usually, a lack of understanding about the topic, so here you go. There are two variants of cholesterol – LDL (low-density lipoprotein) and HDL (high-density lipoprotein). LDL is the so-called "bad" cholesterol because it tends to accumulate in your artery walls, causing them to narrow and escalating the risk of heart disease. On the flip side, HDL is the "good" cholesterol, playing the role of health crusader by ferrying LDL away from the arteries and back to the liver, where it's broken down and evicted from the body (CDC, n.d.).

Imagine LDL as the sticky muck clogging up your arteries, with HDL swooping in as the super cleanser to save the day. And, as with any good superhero tale, you want a battalion of the good guys (HDL) and fewer villains (LDL) to maintain harmony and shield your heart from the dark side. Okay, no more Star Wars references. (I did it for my son-in-law Jason, who is an avid fan and collector of memorabilia).

SETTING THE BAR FOR HEALTHY CHOLESTEROL LEVELS

Now that we've cracked the code on the difference between the "good guys" and the "bad guys" in the cholesterol universe, it's time to understand what constitutes healthy levels. The American Heart Association gives us a neat set of guidelines for cholesterol levels for adults:

- Total cholesterol: Aim for less than 200 mg/dL (milligrams per deciliter). That's the sweet spot.
- LDL cholesterol: Under 100 mg/dL is the golden standard.
- HDL cholesterol: Anything 60 mg/dL or higher is your shield against heart disease.

However, let's not forget that these are just ballpark figures. Individual factors like age, gender, and family history can swing the pendulum on what's optimal for you. As always, it's smart to team up with your healthcare professional to pinpoint the targets that best suit your unique circumstances.

THE LINK BETWEEN CHOLESTEROL AND HEART DISEASE

You might be wondering, why all this aggravation about cholesterol levels? Here's the scoop. When the "bad guys," aka LDL cholesterol levels, skyrocket, they can form a sticky substance known as plaque in your arteries. Over time, this plaque can clog up, stiffen, and narrow your arteries, a pesky condition we call atherosclerosis. When this happens in the coronary arteries, the ones responsible for sending blood to your heart, it can lead to coronary artery disease. This escalates the risk of heart attacks, stroke, and other heart-related complications.

On the flip side, the "good guys," higher levels of HDL cholesterol are like the protectors of your body. They're associated with a lower risk of heart disease because they act like a cleanup crew, escorting LDL cholesterol out of the arteries and preventing plaque formation. Therefore, keeping a healthy balance between LDL and HDL cholesterol is your secret weapon in shielding your heart from heart disease.

STRATEGIES TO MANAGE YOUR CHOLESTEROL LEVELS

Before you resign yourself to a lifetime of celery sticks and rice cakes, or seeds and twigs, let's set the record straight: living a heart-healthy lifestyle doesn't mean you have to banish all your favorite foods. A few smart tweaks to your diet can make a world of difference when it comes to looking after your ticker and managing your cholesterol levels. It has been recommended to me to use the 80/20 rule. 80% of your diet should be as healthy as you can realistically manage. 20% of your diet can be some cheat food. Just don't binge on it or you will defeat all the hard work you accomplish 80% of the time. Bottom line, it has to be manageable for you. Here's the low-down on some simple dietary adjustments that can help keep your heart dancing to the right beat:

1. Choose your meats wisely: Not all meats are created equal. Lean cuts are your heart's best friend, while processed meats like hot dogs and sausages, (sorry),

loaded with unhealthy fats and sodium, are its nemesis. Make that rib-eye a weekend treat. However, if you happen to be in Boston at a Red Sox game, have a Fenway Frank. They're the best.

2. Get choosy with fats: Speaking of fats, remember they're not all bad. In fact, healthy fats, like those found in avocados, nuts, and seeds, are a boon. But saturated and trans fats, hiding in fried foods and packaged snacks, are a curse. So, be selective.

3. Embrace fiber: Soluble fiber, found in foods like oats, beans, and fruits, can help lower LDL cholesterol levels. So, ditch the sugar-packed, processed fodder the marketing industry tries to sell you.

4. Welcome fish into your diet: Fish like salmon, mackerel, and sardines are rich in omega-3 fatty acids and can help reduce your risk of heart disease. Remember, as the movie said, fish are friends... and also food.

5. Master the art of portion control: Even the healthiest foods can do more harm than good if you overindulge. Keep a keen eye on portion sizes and resist the temptation to upsize your meals.

While the allure of Sundays on the couch, or reruns of *Gilligan's Island* can be strong, remember this: your heart loves a good workout. Regular exercise isn't just about keeping your weight in check; it also does wonders for your cholesterol levels by pumping up the HDL and bringing down the LDL. Don't worry if you're not into marathon running or powerlifting. Even small bouts of activity, like taking the stairs or dancing while doing the dishes, can make a world of difference. (And if you do break into a salsa at the sink, do us a favor and make a video, will you?)

You've probably heard the saying "stress can kill," right? Well, there's more than a smidgeon of truth to it. Chronic stress can be a silent saboteur, sneaking up on your blood pressure and cholesterol levels; but there are plenty of healthy ways to tackle stress. Whether it's mindfulness, yoga, or immersing yourself in a hobby, finding your personal Zen can be a shield for your heart. If you golf like me, I don't recommend it for stress reduction.

And let's not forget some other crucial elements of heart health: kicking the smoking habit, reining in the alcohol, and getting a good night's sleep. Each of these steps is like a piece of the puzzle in controlling your cholesterol levels and ensuring your heart stays fit and strong.

A BRIEF OVERVIEW OF HEART DISEASE

It's not just one specific condition, but rather a sneaky assortment of conditions that target your ticker. Here are some of the usual suspects:

1. *Coronary artery disease*: Picture your heart as a city, and the arteries are the highways bringing in essential supplies. When these highways get narrowed or blocked due to a plaque traffic jam, we call it coronary artery disease.
2. *Heart failure*: Don't let the name fool you – it doesn't mean your heart has quit on you completely. Instead, it's like your heart is underperforming on the job, struggling to pump blood as efficiently as it should.

This leads to a fluid buildup in the lungs and other parts of the body.

3. *Arrhythmia*: This is when your heart decides to freestyle its rhythm, beating too fast, too slow, or just plain irregularly – like it's trying to improvise a jazz solo. Atrial fibrillation is one such unpleasant rhythm.

4. *Valvular heart disease*: This happens when one or more of your heart's valves, the gatekeepers of blood flow, are damaged or not functioning correctly.

Symptoms of heart disease come in many shapes and sizes, ranging from chest pain and shortness of breath to palpitations and fatigue. If any of these signs start knocking on your door, do not ignore them. Reach out to a healthcare professional, preferably a Cardiologist or Electro-Physiologist for further evaluation (CDC, n.d.), because when it comes to heart disease, knowledge is the first step to taking control.

These are some of the typical suspects that increase the risk of developing heart disease. Here's the lineup:

1. *High blood pressure*: This forces your heart to work overtime, causing it to tire out faster.

2. *High cholesterol levels*: cholesterol can secretly build up in your arteries, leading to blockages.

3. *Diabetes*: Diabetes and heart disease often go hand in hand causing havoc.

4. *Obesity*: Extra weight makes your heart work harder, and it's not a fan of the extra workload.

5. *Family history of heart disease*: Sometimes, the risk runs in the family.

6. *Smoking*: Your heart doesn't appreciate the smoke. It causes damage to your blood vessels, increasing your risk.
7. *Unhealthy diet*: Too much salt, fat, and sugar in your diet can lead to high blood pressure and cholesterol.
8. *Physical inactivity*: Not getting up and moving enough can make your heart rusty and underperforming.
9. *Age*: Like a vintage car, the heart will start having more issues as it ages.
10. *Gender*: Men tend to be at higher risk, but ladies, don't let your guard down. After menopause, your risk increases too.

While some of these risk factors, like your age and family history, are non-negotiable, there are many that you have power over. Making lifestyle changes can significantly reduce your risk, turning the tables on heart disease. However, there is a balance between genetics and lifestyle when it comes to heart disease. The scenario is a high-stakes game of cards. Genetics is the hand you're dealt at birth. You have no control over it. It could be a royal flush or a dud. Now, lifestyle is how you play that hand, and that is entirely up to you.

Having a family history of heart disease might mean your hand is not the best. But you can trump that genetic predisposition with a lifestyle that can be "heart healthy." It's all about finding the right balance. Making modifications can dramatically lower your risk of developing heart disease, even if your genes are trying to lead you down that path. Now, it's your turn to show it some love. It takes patience and persistence.

To get an idea of what your heart does in a lifetime, look at these rough estimates for a 60-to-70-year-old man: Let's assume a resting heart rate of 70 beats per minute. Calculate the number of beats in a year. That's 36,792,000 beats/year. So, based on these assumptions, the average 60-to-70-year-old man would have approximately 2,759,400,000 beats in his lifetime. That dude has done some work, all on your behalf.

PREVENTING HEART DISEASE – PROACTIVE STEPS

Adopting a heart-conscious lifestyle may initially seem like an ambitious endeavor. However, in reality, it unfolds more like an intentional process marked by thoughtful, daily decisions that contribute to a wide-ranging strategy for heart health. Importantly, this proactive approach not only strengthens your heart but also promotes overall health.

First and foremost, nutrition plays a pivotal role in heart health. As I've covered before, a well-balanced diet serves as the foundation for maintaining optimal cholesterol levels and preventing inflammatory processes that could potentially harm your cardiovascular system. The incorporation of beneficial fats found in nuts, seeds, and certain types of fish, for instance, can help lower low-density lipoprotein cholesterol – often referred to as "bad cholesterol" – and mitigate inflammation.

Physical activity, another critical pillar of heart health, doesn't necessitate arduous training or countless hours spent in the gym. The goal is to find a form of exercise that you enjoy and can maintain consistently, thereby making heart health not just a health requirement (AHA, n.d.), but also a fulfilling aspect of your lifestyle.

MEDICAL SCREENING AND PROMPT DETECTION

The adage, "Prevention is better than cure," holds substantial truth, particularly in the territory of heart health. Regular medical examinations and appropriate screening tests provide a strong defense against cardiovascular diseases, enabling early detection and mitigation of risk factors.

Routine monitoring of cholesterol and blood pressure levels is indispensable, along with any additional tests your healthcare provider may suggest. Particularly, if your family history reveals an increased predisposition to heart disease, you may require more frequent evaluations. I, too, have been guilty of not getting tests, even when I've been "enthusiastically encouraged" by my wife. I have good friends who think it's a scam – "All they want is more and more tests." Though there are a few unprincipled people in the medical community, the vast majority want to see you get and stay healthy. It's critical to engage in open conversations with your doctor about your potential risk factors to ensure a tailored and effective preventive strategy.

KEY TAKEAWAYS

1. Understanding cholesterol and its impact on heart health is crucial for preventing heart disease.
2. A heart-healthy lifestyle includes a balanced diet, regular exercise, and stress management.
3. Regular medical screenings and early detection can play a significant role in maintaining good heart health.
4. Heart disease prevention is possible through proactive steps and overall wellness.

FINAL THOUGHTS

The power to safeguard your heart and keep it robust for the long haul lies in your hands. By realizing cholesterol's role, embracing a heart-nurturing lifestyle, and being proactive about screenings for early detection, you're steering your own fate. Don't let heart disease call the shots for your future. Grab the chance to implement meaningful changes and welcome a life full of energy and wellness.

As we step into the next chapter, we'll investigate another crucial component of men's health: the prostate. Just as your heart does, your prostate demands care and vigilance to ensure a vibrant and healthy life. Let's continue on toward peak wellness by understanding how to defend and sustain this essential organ.

13

MAKING SENSE OF YOUR PROSTATE – AN INSIGHTFUL EXPLORATION

To understand why prostate health is so crucial, we must first get to know our little friend. The prostate is a small, walnut-sized gland located just below the bladder and in front of the rectum. It's an essential part of the male reproductive system, responsible for producing a fluid that mixes with sperm to create semen.

But that's not all. The prostate also has a few other responsibilities, like helping to control the flow of urine and playing a role in sexual response. So, it's safe to say that this little powerhouse has a lot on its plate.

COMMON PROSTATE PROBLEMS AND SYMPTOMS

Now that we've had a meet-and-greet with our silent hero, let's talk about some of the issues that can arise when it's not performing at its best. Here are a few common prostate pitfalls:

- *Prostatitis:* Picture a storm brewing, right there in your prostate. It is an inflammation or infection of the prostate gland that that translates into a hell of a lot of pain, difficulty urinating, and sometimes fever. While it's usually not life-threatening, it can be pretty darn uncomfortable.
- *Benign Prostatic Hyperplasia (BPH):* As men get on in years, our prostate decides to take up a new hobby: it grows, and sometimes, like a zucchini in your garden, it gets a bit overzealous, leading to BPH. Symptoms? A bladder with a mind of its own, including frequent urges, weak flow, and difficulty starting and stopping. Another thrill and joy of aging. Your chance of having BPH increase with age:
- Age 31-40: one in 12
- Age 51-60: about one in 2
- Over age 80: more than eight in 10
- *Prostate Cancer:* This is the big one. Prostate cancer is the second most common cancer in men worldwide. It can often be asymptomatic in its early stages, quiet, like a church mouse, but as it progresses, it may cause symptoms similar to BPH, as well as blood in the urine or semen, and pain in the lower back, hips, or thighs (National Cancer Institute, n.d.). According to the American Cancer Society, most cases of prostate cancer can't be prevented, mostly because its causes are still unknown.

So, having seen the threat of these potential dangers, it's glaringly obvious that prostate care isn't something to be shrugged off or pushed to the back burner. On the contrary, it's a red-alert necessity. Being on the front foot about prostate health isn't just a good idea – it's an absolute must. After all, it plays a feature role in your overall well-being and the quality of your daily life.

Keeping your prostate in great shape is a bit like carrying an insurance policy against these troubles. It helps keep them at bay, or at least catch them while they're still a manageable issues rather than a full-blown disaster. And hey, who wouldn't want to safeguard their sex life and urinary expertise – two aspects of manhood we're pretty darn attached to.

Prostate health isn't just another box to tick on your health checklist, it's non-negotiable. It's a mission, should you choose to accept, about being the best man you can be, for yourself and for those you love.

STRATEGIES TO KEEP YOUR PROSTATE IN FIGHTING FORM

Now, let's talk about some battle strategies for your prostate, starting with the biggie: your plate. What you shovel into your mouth is as important as your exercise routine when it comes to keeping your prostate firing on all cylinders. A balanced, nutritious diet is your secret weapon for maintaining not just your prostate, but your overall health. And, lucky for us, there are some foods that are like a love letter to your prostate.

Diet and nutrition for a healthy prostate

Let's start with the basics. Fruits and veggies are your new best friends, especially the ones that are chock-full of antioxidants. Take tomatoes, for instance. They're full of lycopene, an antioxidant that's like a knight in shining armor for your prostate. Also, give a standing ovation to cruciferous veggies like broccoli, cauliflower, and cabbage - they've been known to pack a punch against cancer (JNCI, 2003).

And let's not forget the fat. The good kind, of course. Nuts, seeds, and fatty fish are brimming with healthy fats. Omega-3 fatty acids are the stars of the show here, as they've been linked to a lower risk of prostate cancer.

And last but not least, embrace whole grains and legumes. They're fiber powerhouses, which is a surefire way to keep your prostate grinning from ear to ear. Just remember, everything in moderation. Try to resist the siren call of red and processed meats. They might taste good, but they're not doing your prostate any favors.

So, there you have it, gentlemen. Fuel your body with the good stuff, and you'll be doing your prostate – and yourself – a huge favor. Happy eating!

THE ROLE OF PHYSICAL ACTIVITY AND EXERCISE

Ready to pound the pavement, or at least the treadmill? Because it turns out that working up a sweat is a big thumbs up not just for your waistline, but also for your prostate. Consistent physical activity has been connected with a lower chance of your prostate throwing a tantrum in the form of prostate cancer or other related issues. Plus, exercise is like a vitamin shot for your overall health, making it a double whammy of benefits. Your mission, a minimum of 30 minutes of moderate-intensity aerobic exercise. Taking a very a brisk walk or a bike ride that gets your heart pumping, even a swim that leaves you feeling invigorated on most days of the week. And of course, strength training, it's like the secret sauce to maintaining your muscle mass and keeping your metabolism purring like a well-tuned engine.

THE TWISTY MAZE OF PROSTATE CANCER – RISKS AND HOW TO DODGE 'EM

Prostate cancer is a bit like your first serious relationship: it's complicated. There are multiple factors that color the picture, some of which are, age, race, and family history, and those aren't exactly something with which you can negotiate. Don't throw in the towel just yet. There are other factors you can change, like diet, exercise, and lifestyle choices, which can influence your risk of prostate cancer.

Now, here's the thing about prostate cancer: it's got a bit of a Dr. Jekyll and Mr. Hyde thing going on. It can be a real gentleman if you catch it early. More treatment options, better chances of sending it packing for good. That's why regular check-ups are your secret weapon here.

The current and best strategy suggests you start discussing prostate cancer screenings with your doctor when you hit 50. If you've got a family history or belong to a higher-risk group, you might want to start that conversation earlier. You're probably in line for a digital rectal exam (DRE) and a prostate-specific antigen test (PSA). However, the PSA test, which is often used to screen for prostate cancer, has been a bit of a hot potato. It's been known to lead to overdiagnosis and overtreatment. So, it's crucial to have a heart-to-heart with your healthcare provider to weigh up the pros and cons and figure out the best game plan for you (American Cancer Society, n.d.).

While you can't exactly tell "Father Time" to take a hike or pick your family tree, there are plenty of proactive steps you can take to lower your risk of prostate cancer. By opting for a healthier lifestyle, you can decrease your chances of crossing paths with prostate problems and give your overall health a major boost. It's not just about fighting the good fight; it's about winning it!

Here is your playbook for outsmarting prostate cancer:

1. Commandeer the kitchen. Fill your plate with a colorful array of fruits, vegetables, whole grains, and the good kind of fats.
2. Get your sweat on regularly, with a combination of aerobic and strength training exercises. If it gets your heart pumping and your muscles flexing, you're on the right track.
3. Keep stress in check. Discover the Zen-like bliss of relaxation techniques, meditation, or yoga. They're like kryptonite for stress.
4. Prioritize sleep and stick to a consistent bedtime routine. It's not just for kids, you know.
5. Give smoking the boot and keep a tight rein on alcohol. Your prostate will thank you.

These lifestyle tweaks won't just help you with prevention of prostate cancer, they'll also give your overall health a shot in the arm. Taking the reins of your health isn't just liberating; it's a game-changer. By making these positive shifts, you're not just making a one-off investment. Ready to take the plunge?

KEY TAKEAWAYS

- Your prostate is a crucial part of your body, and maintaining its health is essential for your overall well-being.
- A healthy lifestyle, including a balanced diet, regular exercise, and stress management, can help keep your prostate in good shape and lower your risk of developing issues.
- Understanding your risk factors for prostate cancer and being proactive with screening and checkups can lead to early detection and more effective treatment.
- Taking control of your prostate health is an investment in your future and can significantly impact your quality of life.

FINAL THOUGHTS

We've taken a deep dive into the world of prostate health in this chapter, unearthing the importance of this powerhouse gland and the measures you can take to keep it running smoothly. The risk of prostate issues might seem like a steep mountain to climb, but remember this: Knowledge is your climbing gear, and being proactive about your health is your guide up the mountain.

You're now equipped with several tools and intel you need to take charge of your prostate health, empowering you to chart a course toward positive changes that will benefit your overall well-being. As you continue your venture toward a healthier, happier life, remember to keep prostate health in the passenger seat, and your body will be thanking you down the road.

As we tie a bow on this chapter, let's clear the stage for our next act: the all-important subject of your sexual health and its role in your overall wellness. In our next chapter, we'll unravel the essential role sexual health plays in our lives and offer strategies for achieving and maintaining its fitness.

14

THE METHOD AND SCIENCE OF SEXUAL HEALTH – MASTERING THE DANCE

Y ou're kicked back in your favorite armchair, a peaceful evening unfurling around you. Your mind wanders down memory lane, back to the days when you were a spry young buck, brimming with enthusiasm and vitality. As your thoughts roam, you ponder your love life's trajectory and how it has morphed over the years. A question nudges its way to the forefront of your mind, "Is this it? Is this the sunset of my virility?" Whoa, hold your horses, compadre! You're not the Lone Ranger on this quest for enlightenment, there are folks here, me included, to help you navigate the often cryptic and clandestine domain of sexual health in the autumn of life.

In this chapter, we're going to plunge headfirst into the science behind the metamorphosis in sexual health as you saunter down the path of life. We'll shatter some myths and misconceptions and arm you with the toolkit you need to super-charge your testosterone and preserve a robust and fulfilling love life.

YOUR SEXUAL LIFE AS YOU AGE

As we gather more candles on our birthday cakes, our bodies decide to throw us a few curveballs. Not just those sly silver strands making their way into your hair or those stubborn lines that seem to etch themselves deeper on your face with each passing year. It goes deeper, quite literally. Hormone levels decide to dance to their own tune, muscles start to slack off a bit, and the plumbing may not be as lively as it once was. But that's not the end of it! Your mental and emotional state decides to join the party and influence your sexual well-being. You might notice your libido deciding to take a vacation, anxiety levels creeping up, or self-awareness turning up a notch, even feelings of inadequacy or embarrassment making unwanted guest appearances. While these changes might be part and parcel of our aging, they don't necessarily have to sound the death knell for your love life.

As our vintage gets more vintager, it's not uncommon to experience a variety of sexual challenges. For men, erectile dysfunction (ED) might be at the top of the list, affecting an estimated 50% of men over the age of 40. Don't panic! This statistic isn't meant to scare you but to illustrate that ED is a common issue that many men face as they age (Mayo Clinic, n.d.). I believe the percentage is higher, but most men are resistant to divulge that type of personal information. That alone should tell you that when it comes to our health, our ego must leave the room. Call him back when the conversation is over.

Other speed bumps you might come across include a dip in sexual desire, challenges in scoring or sustaining an erection, and alterations in orgasm or ejaculation. Ladies, meanwhile, might grapple with vaginal dryness, a dwindling libido, or discomfort during lovemaking. But don't lose heart! There's a veritable smorgasbord of solutions and strategies up for grabs to help navigate these challenges and keep your love life humming.

ADDRESSING THE ELEPHANT IN THE ROOM

Our society seems to have developed some, let's say, "interesting" notions about sex and aging. But the truth is, you can continue to lead a spiced-up and fulfilling sex life well into your senior years.

Myth 1: Sex is a playground exclusive to the spring chickens.
Busted! Sex is a natural and pleasurable facet of life, open to all age brackets. In fact, studies reveal that older adults who keep the home fires burning report higher levels of happiness and well-being compared to their less active counterparts.

Myth 2: A hibernating sex life equals poor health. Misguided! There's a whole gamut of factors that can impact a person's sex life, including health conditions, medications, and emotional state. A decline in sexual activity doesn't necessarily paint you as unhealthy; it's more a signal that you might need to tweak a few things or seek medical advice to address any underlying issues.

*Myth 3: Reach a certain age, and your sex drive decides to up and leave.*Incorrect! While it's true that hormonal shifts can play a role in your libido, it doesn't necessarily sign you up for a lifetime membership to the "no-sex club." Plenty of older adults continue to enjoy active and gratifying sex lives, even if the frequency or intensity might take on a new rhythm over time.

Myth 4: Erectile dysfunction is an accepted guest at the aging party. While it's accurate that ED tends to show up more often as men age, it's not an unchangeable part of the script. ED can be influenced by a variety of factors, including health conditions, medications, and lifestyle choices. Addressing these underlying issues can often help bring back the spark in erectile function.

Myth 5: Are you stuck with age-related sexual challenges? Absolutely not! There's an entire toolkit of strategies, treatments, and lifestyle shifts that can help navigate sexual challenges and keep the flame alive in your sex life as you age. So, don't throw in the towel – stick with me, and we'll explore the solutions and resources at your disposal to tackle these issues head-on.

TESTOSTERONE AND ITS ROLE IN SEXUAL HEALTH

Testosterone. Often typecast as the "male hormone," it's crucial to the sexual health and overall well-being of both men and women. It's the mastermind behind a host of biological functions, including bulking up muscle mass, maintaining bone density, orchestrating facial and body hair growth, and, of course, fueling the sex drive. For men, the testicles are the primary production house of testosterone, while in women, the ovaries take on this role (albeit in much smaller quantities).

Much like the perfectly ripe avocado at the grocery store, testosterone levels hit their prime in our youth and start to descend as we age. This is a natural part of life's rhythm, typically kicking off in men around 30 and continuing at a pace of roughly 1% per year (Manual, n.d.). However, some men may experience a more dramatic plunge in testosterone levels, leading to a condition known as hypogonadism or the less scary sounding "low T."

Low T doesn't just impact your sex life – it can have far-reaching consequences for your overall health and well-being. Some common symptoms of low testosterone include low sex drive, erectile dysfunction, fatigue, muscle weakness, and even mood changes like irritability or depression. Additionally, low T can increase your risk of developing other health issues, such as osteoporosis and cardiovascular disease. Many men are turning to TRT, testosterone replacement therapy. Following is a list of ways TRT can help not only our sexual health, but our overall health as well:

- *Increased energy levels*: TRT can boost energy levels, reducing fatigue and enhancing overall vitality.
- *Improved mood*: TRT may alleviate symptoms of depression, irritability, and mood swings, leading to an improved sense of well-being.
- *Enhanced sexual function*: TRT can help improve libido, erectile function, and sexual satisfaction.
- *Increased muscle mass and strength*: TRT can facilitate muscle growth and strength development, aiding in physical performance and exercise outcomes.
- *Reduced body fat*: TRT may contribute to the reduction of excess body fat, particularly in the abdominal region.

- *Increased bone density*: TRT can improve bone mineral density, reducing the risk of osteoporosis and fractures.
- *Improved cognitive function*: TRT might enhance cognitive abilities such as memory, focus, and concentration.
- *Increased red blood cell production*: TRT can stimulate the production of red blood cells, potentially improving oxygen delivery throughout the body.
- *Better cardiovascular health*: TRT may have a positive impact on heart health by reducing the risk of cardiovascular diseases.
- *Restored sleep patterns*: TRT might help improve sleep quality and alleviate sleep disturbances, leading to better rest and recovery.

The benefits of TRT can vary depending on individual circumstances, and it is important to discuss this therapy with your doctor for tailored advice and treatment that meets your specific needs.

STRATEGIES TO KEEP THE SPARKS FLYING AS YOU AGE

Let's Talk About It – Communication and Intimacy with Your Better Half

As the years pile on, the importance of keeping a heart-to-heart connection with your partner skyrockets. By opening up about your sexual aspirations, worries, and stumbling blocks, you'll both get a better grasp of each other's needs, creating a closeness and connection that can't be beat. The birds and bees talk shouldn't be a one-hit-wonder – it should be a chart-topping hit on repeat! Remember, the ride to a satisfying sex life is a tandem bicycle, not a solo sprint!

New Tricks for Old Dogs – Exploring Different Avenues of Pleasure

Whoever said you can't teach an old dog new tricks haven't met you! As Father Time does his thing, it's crucial to keep an open mind and be game for discovering different ways to light the fire of pleasure. This could mean trying out new positions that don't require a gymnast's flexibility, bringing toys or lubricants into the mix, or indulging in non-penetrative fun, like sensual massages or oral play. The aim of the game is to mix it up and keep the novelty alive – who knows, you might stumble upon a new bedroom favorite!

Tackling Health Issues that Impact Your Sex Life

With the march of time, our bodies become more prone to health hiccups that can throw a wrench in the gears of our sexual function. If you find yourself wrestling with challenges like erectile dysfunction or a waning libido, it's time to rally the troops and seek professional advice. Your healthcare provider can help pinpoint any underlying health gremlins and recommend possible treatments, like medication or hormone replacement therapy, to help you reclaim your mojo. I have stated that I have a disdain for the influence Big Pharma has over many aspects of our lives. But the research that has been accomplished because of their influence/profits have allowed for an untold number of chemical compounds that enhance, protect, and save millions of lives. Medications in and of themselves are not bad, it's the over reliance on them that perpetuates ill health in many. If everything you have tried does not address the root cause of your affliction, then it's off to the pharmacy, with my blessing. (See Chapter 2, RCA)

HEALTHY LIVING FOR A HEALTHY LOVING – THE ROLE OF LIFESTYLE

A healthy sex life is built on the bedrock of a healthy lifestyle, regardless of how many candles are on your birthday cake. Actively prioritizing your physical, mental, and emotional well-being can do wonders for your sexual prowess. This includes fueling your body with a balanced diet, keeping active, nailing stress management, getting enough sleep, and steering clear of excessive boozing or smoking. And remember, it's never too late to make changes for the better – even baby steps can lead to giant leaps in your overall health and sex life.

Aging doesn't have to mean putting the brakes on your sex life. By staying in the know, keeping the lines of communication with your partner open, and proactively addressing any concerns about your sexual health, you can continue to enjoy a satisfying and fulfilling sex life well into your sunset years.

So, embrace the wisdom that comes with age, and enjoy your sex life with your partner.

Here are a couple tips to maintain a healthy sex life

Stay active, engage in regular exercise, and eat a balanced diet – these will make a significant difference in most every area of your life. Do your best to manage your stress and make self-care a priority in your life – you're worth it. Seek medical help when it's necessary – sometimes our bodies need a little extra help to keep "stuff" moving correctly. Lastly, what are you waiting for? Go live your life!

KEY TAKEAWAYS

- Open communication with your partner and exploring new ways to experience pleasure can help maintain a healthy sex life as you age.
- Regular exercise, a balanced diet, and stress management are essential components of a sexually satisfying lifestyle.
- Low testosterone levels can impact sexual health and overall well-being, but treatments like testosterone replacement therapy can provide relief.
- Seeking medical help when faced with sexual health challenges is crucial for maintaining a fulfilling sex life.

FINAL THOUGHTS

As you work your way through the winding path of life, it's key to remember that your sexual health is a major player on your team. Welcome the changes that come hand-in-hand with aging and meet any hurdles head-on with a proactive spirit. By taking the reins of your health, keeping the conversation flowing with your partner, and continually seeking new paths to pleasure, you can keep the flame of a fulfilling sex life burning bright well into your twilight years. There's no time like the present to prioritize and invest in your sexual well-being – because you deserve a life rich with passion, intimacy, and joy, no matter how many rings you've added to your tree of life.

In the upcoming chapter, I will tap into the world of cognitive health and how to keep all that gray matter in your cranium on full throttle as you age.

15

PREVENTATIVE MEASURES

R egardless of your current position in life's grand tapestry, the opportunity to take the reins on your future health status is yours for the taking. Indeed, it's time to translate the amassed wisdom into action and get the ball rolling. We're sounding the bugle for today.

This short chapter serves as your compass toward achieving success by implementing preemptive measures. So, gather together all the pearls of wisdom you've collected on your way and plunge into the depths of preventive healthcare. Something I believe many insurance companies are finally seeing as valuable.

THE GRAVITY OF HEALTHY AGING

By this point, you should have a good grasp of the profound significance that healthy aging carries. It's not just about bearing the semblance of a timeless Adonis as the sands of time slip away (although that's certainly an enticing side-benefit); it's about a profound sense of wellness and the realization of a life packed with rich experiences. You should realize that healthy aging improves the odds of retaining your autonomy, evading the snares of chronic ailments, and preserving the passion to enjoy the many things that make your heart keep beating.

Preventive measures play the role of a covert mixture in the context of healthy aging. They pivot around the viewpoint of nourishing your body and soul in the present to savor in the prospect of health in the future. This necessitates an active commitment to your physical, mental, and emotional well-being, coupled with the resolution to address up-and-coming issues before they mushroom into serious predicaments. So, while the quest for a mythical fountain of youth might be a fool's errand (sorry, gentlemen), preventive measures are the closest approximation you've got.

ANOTHER VISIT TO YOUR ROADBLOCKS

It's time to uncover what's stalling your road to a healthier life. Are you seduced by midnight pizza raids? Whatever it may be, it's crucial to pinpoint the root cause or causes of these unhealthy patterns.

To kick off, arm yourself with the accompanying journal and jot down anything you suspect might be your roadblock. Be frank with yourself, and don't shy away from some honest answers. Don't forget, this isn't a judgment zone – it's all about self-growth!

With your health hurdles laid out, it's time to strategize. Think like a chess grandmaster and plan your winning moves. For each obstruction you've listed, write out some possible solutions. If you're prone to nocturnal nibbling, for instance, consider trading junk food for healthier alternatives.

Remember, surmounting obstacles requires time and effort, so if the results aren't immediate, don't beat yourself up. This is all about gradual, manageable tweaks that build up to make a huge difference over time.

A MOTIVATION MIND HACK

Have you ever considered that your brain is essentially your very own motivational coach? Remember Dopamine? Each time you score a goal, your brain rewards you by releasing that wonder drug to create a delightful, satisfying sensation. It functions as a motivational award, sparking you to continue striving and tackling further obstacles. So, how can you trick your mind into releasing more? Initiate by setting minor, achievable goals. Each of these small victories will trigger a hit of dopamine, nudging you forward on your journey to a healthier lifestyle.

Techniques to cultivate a growth mindset

The growth mindset is like motivation's secret weapon. It revolves around the belief that your skills can be honed and amplified through hard work and persistence. In essence, it's the conviction that you can indeed teach an old dog new tricks.

To develop this growth mindset, consider these techniques:

- *Embrace obstacles*: Rather than sidestepping hardships, perceive them as opportunities to expand and acquire knowledge.

- *Learn from mistakes*: It's an integral part of the journey. Treat your missteps as invaluable lessons guiding you toward triumph.
- *Value effort*: Understand that commitment and hard work are the real catalysts of growth, not just inborn talent.
- *Welcome feedback*: Constructive criticism can aid in spotting areas ripe for growth, so refrain from taking it to heart. Instead, use it as kindling for self-improvement.

OLD HABITS ARE VERY CLINGY

Breaking old habits can feel like an uphill battle – they didn't earn the name "habits" for nothing. However, the bright side is, it's entirely possible to swap those less-than-healthy routines with new, better ones. Here are some strategies to help you:

- *Spot your triggers*: Identify what cues or circumstances kickstart your unhealthy habits, then strategize on how to sidestep or handle them.
- *Substitute, not obliterate*: Rather than striving to entirely annihilate a bad habit, focus on exchanging it for a healthier option. For instance, replace your afternoon chocolate bar with a juicy apple.
- *Begin modestly*: Avoid the urge to revamp your whole lifestyle in a day. Concentrate instead on making one tiny adjustment at a time, using each success as a steppingstone.

Creating a bearable healthy lifestyle hinges on instilling

enduring changes that eventually become innate. For this to happen, consistency in practicing your new habits is key, coupled with patience as you adapt. Keep in mind, establishing new routines takes time, so hold off on expecting instantaneous results. And, most critically, extend some compassion to yourself throughout the process. Also, everyone has a unique timetable for adopting a new routine in their lives. You'll know when it's yours.

THE FUNDAMENTALS TO NOT BECOMING "SOME OLD DUDE"

Some would call it, "The Essentials of Healthy Aging." You've heard it a million times before, but it bears repeating: exercise, proper nutrition, and sufficient sleep are the holy trinity of healthy aging. Together, they form the foundation for a vibrant, energetic, and disease-free life. Plus, they make you look and feel like a million bucks.

Here are some tips to help you get started:

1. *Find an exercise routine you enjoy*: Whether it's dancing, swimming, or taking long walks in the park, pick an activity that makes you happy and gets your heart pumping.
2. *Make it social*: Enlist a workout buddy or join a group class to make exercise more fun and increase accountability. After all, misery loves company, and so does a good sweat session!
3. *Plan your meals*: Take some time each week to plan out your meals and snacks, focusing on a balanced diet

full of fruits, veggies, lean proteins, and whole grains. This will make it easier to stick to healthy eating habits and avoid impulsive junk food binges.

4. *Prioritize sleep*: Treat yourself to a regular sleep schedule and create a bedtime routine that signals to your body that it's time to wind down. This might include reading, meditating, or enjoying a warm cup of herbal tea. Oh, and maybe skip that late-night horror movie marathon – your sleep (and sanity) will thank you.

5. *Be flexible*: Life happens, and sometimes your plans for a healthy lifestyle might get derailed. The key is to be adaptable and get back on track as soon as you can. Remember, progress, not perfection, is the goal.

There you have it – the secret recipe for hacking your mind, breaking old habits, and incorporating the essentials of healthy aging into your daily life. By embracing these strategies, you'll be well on your way to a brighter, more vibrant, and healthier future.

And remember, the biggest, often the hardest thing is to just get started. Start slow if you need to, but get started. Learning to be healthy can help you live the best life possible.

DISEASE MITIGATION

Here are some crucial pointers to help you fend off those irritating age-related diseases. Stay on top of recommended vaccines to safeguard against flu, pneumonia, shingles, and other age-associated illnesses.

- *Make your doctor a close ally*: Regular health checkups are paramount for detecting potential health problems early on. Keep an eye on your numbers: Monitor your blood pressure, cholesterol, and blood sugar levels. These numbers serve as your health's vital signs, and being aware of them can guide you in making informed lifestyle choices.

- *Laugh stress away:* While not necessarily in a literal sense, finding healthy stress management techniques can significantly affect your overall health. It's crucial to remember that maintaining top-notch health isn't a one-off endeavor; it's a continual excursion that demands constant vigilance and adaptation. Like a well-tuned machine, your body needs regular upkeep to function optimally.

Here are some other tips to keep you ahead in your health quest:

- *Tune in to your body:* Your body has a knack for alerting you when something's off. Stay vigilant for any changes in how you feel and don't hesitate to reach out to a healthcare professional if something seems unusually amiss. Stay in the loop: Keep abreast with the latest health news and research. Knowledge is indeed power, and staying informed empowers you to make sound decisions about your health and well-being.

- *Be flexible:* As you age, your body's requirements will shift. Be open to adjusting your lifestyle, exercise regimen, and dietary habits to accommodate these changes and persist in prioritizing your health.

PUTTING IT ALL TOGETHER: CREATING A HOLISTIC HEALTHY LIFESTYLE

Now that we've covered a wide range of topics related to healthy aging, it's time to put all that information to good use. Think of this as a puzzle, and each chapter represents a piece that, when combined, creates a complete picture of a healthy, fulfilling life.

To create your personalized plan for healthy aging, consider the following steps:

- Reflect on the lessons learned throughout this book and identify the areas where you'd like to see improvement in your life.
- Set realistic, achievable goals for yourself in each area, remembering to focus on progress rather than perfection.
- Break your goals down into smaller, manageable steps, and develop a plan to work on them consistently.
- Regularly evaluate your progress and make adjustments to your plan as needed, ensuring you continue to prioritize your health and well-being.

MISSION: HEALTHY AGING – YOUR PERSONAL BLUEPRINT

Embarking on a quest for healthy aging is an adventure, and like any epic journey, it requires a well-crafted blueprint to guide you along the way. In this section, we present you with "Mission: Healthy Aging," a series of activities designed to help you take immediate action and create long-term goals for sustained well-being. By developing and implementing your personalized action plan, you'll set yourself up for a lifetime of success, conquering the challenges of aging with confidence and grace. Let's dive into the activities that will propel you towards a vibrant, healthy future!

Immediate changes for a healthier life

1. Set an alarm to remind you to take short breaks throughout the day to stretch, walk around, or do a quick workout.
2. Swap out sugary snacks for healthier alternatives like fruit or nuts.
3. Make a commitment to get a full night's sleep by setting a consistent bedtime and creating a relaxing bedtime routine.

Long-term goals for sustained well-being

1. If you're not currently exercising regularly, set a goal to gradually increase your physical activity. Start with short walks or low-impact workouts and work your way up to more challenging routines.

2. Make a plan to incorporate more whole, nutrient-dense foods into your diet, focusing on adding a variety of fruits, vegetables, lean proteins, and whole grains.
3. Prioritize mental health by setting aside time for relaxation, self-care, and stress management activities like meditation or journaling.

KEY TAKEAWAYS

1. Healthy aging involves integrating lessons from various aspects of life, including diet, exercise, mental health, and disease prevention.
2. Regularly monitoring and adapting to your body's changing needs is crucial for maintaining optimal health as you age.
3. Create a personalized plan for healthy aging by setting achievable goals and breaking them down into manageable steps.
4. Immediate changes and long-term goals are both essential for fostering sustained well-being throughout your life.
5. Prioritize your health and well-being by continuously learning, adapting, and making positive lifestyle choices.

FINAL THOUGHTS

As we bring this chapter – and our journey through the world of healthy aging – to a close, it's essential to remember that the power to make positive changes lies within you. It's never too late to start prioritizing your health and well-being, and each small step you take can have a significant impact on your overall quality of life. Embrace the knowledge you've gained, put it into practice, and remember to be patient with yourself as you work toward creating a healthier, happier version of you.

16

"WHEN THE OLD MAN KNOCKS AT THE DOOR, I DON'T LET HIM IN."

Clint Eastwood

The following is an overview of ways to enrich your life and achieve optimal health.

Revamping Your Food Choices:

Consume an abundance of nature's best – a colorful mix of fruits, vegetables, whole grains, lean proteins, and good fats. Supplement your diet with key nutrients like omega-3 fatty acids, readily available in fatty fish like salmon, flaxseeds, and walnuts. Keep a distance from overly processed foods, sugary drink traps, and a high-sodium diet which can wreak havoc on your health.

Cultivating a Fitness Regimen:

Immerse yourself in activities that you enjoy, whether it's swimming laps, cycling, or even breaking a sweat on the dance floor. Integrate strength-training into your fitness plan to bolster muscle strength and bone density – particularly important as we age. Venture into new physical pursuits like yoga or martial arts to improve flexibility and foster a deeper mind-body connection.

Taking Care of Your Mental Fitness:

Harness the power of stress control techniques, such as meditation, deep breathing exercises, or mindfulness – they're not just buzzwords but useful tools in managing mental health. Dedicate time to self-care routines like taking a steam bath, reading a good book, or pursuing your favorite hobbies. Don't shy away from therapy or counseling to tackle emotional issues, past traumas, or unresolved matters – there's strength in seeking help. Achieving equilibrium between work, social engagements, and personal life is paramount for a holistic health strategy.

Setting Your Personal Boundaries:

Master the art of saying "No" when necessary – your time and energy are precious commodities, especially to fend off burnout. Place strict restrictions on work-related tasks, keeping them within set work hours – you've earned your downtime (sometimes easier said than done). Clearly express your need for personal space and time to colleagues, family, and friends.

Finding Relief in Hobbies and Interests:

Many of you have never considered scheduling a dedicated "me time" to indulge in activities that bring you joy and fulfillment, like painting, playing a musical instrument, or even gardening. Do it, get to know yourself, you'll be surprised at your breadth of knowledge and skills. Broaden your horizons by trying out new hobbies or exploring creative outlets to encourage personal growth and self-expression. Join clubs, groups, or community organizations that align with your interests to connect with like-minded peers.

Cultivating Healthy Relationships:

Carve out quality time to connect with your loved ones – schedule regular family meals or date nights with your partner. Keep communication channels open and actively listen to the needs and concerns of your family and friends – relationships need nurturing. Participate in social events or gatherings to build a strong sense of community and belonging.

A well-rounded plan for living your best life should address various aspects of well-being. Here's a three-pronged guide:

Physical Activity and Exercise:

Select activities that you enjoy and are sustainable in the long run – think jogging, hiking, or engaging in team sports, even golf. Incorporate strength training into your regimen to increase muscle mass and overall fitness – it's a proven strategy to combat age-related muscle loss. Set definitive goals – perhaps you'd like to participate in a 10K, complete a challenging hiking trail, or beat your personal bests in certain exercises.

Nutrition:

Make a balanced and bearable diet plan featuring a variety of nutrient-dense foods like leafy greens, whole grains, lean proteins, and good fats. Spice up your meals by experimenting with new recipes and flavors – a healthy diet doesn't have to be dull. Embrace mindful eating – pay attention to hunger cues and savor every bite, every flavor, every texture of your meals.

Self-Care and Stress Management:

Identify effective stress management techniques that resonate with you – yoga, meditation, or journaling may all provide significant benefits. Establish a regular sleep routine – a good night's rest is key to maintaining optimal health and vitality, especially as you age. Carve out time for self-care activities – whether it's a relaxing bath, practicing gratitude, or indulging in a cherished hobby or pastime.

Remember, these guidelines are just a launchpad. Your journey towards optimal health should be tailored to your personal preferences, circumstances, and objectives. After all, you're not just adding years to your life, but life to your years. Sorry for the cliché.

Congratulations! You've navigated to the conclusion of this book, and my sincere hope is that you've found it enlightening, empowering, and even entertaining. I want to halt momentarily to acknowledge the considerable personal transition you're about to undertake.

Change, as we all know, is not for the faint-hearted. It requires courage, tenacity, and steadfast determination. And yet, here you are, ready and willing to commit to a healthier lifestyle that promises to enhance not only your life, but also the lives of those in your circle.

This voyage you're about to set out on is more similar to a marathon than a sprint. There will undoubtedly be setbacks, obstacles, and days when you question the worth of it all. When such moments arise, I encourage you to recall your "why" – why you decided to undertake this commitment in the first place. Think about where you will be a year from right now. Your actions today will determine your future. Make it happen! You are deserving of the time and effort required, and you merit the vibrant and fulfilling existence that comes with improved health and well-being.

As you move forward, make it a point to celebrate the small wins. Maybe it's the first time you ascend a flight of stairs without losing your breath, or the day you realize your favorite pair of jeans fit just perfectly. While these moments may seem trivial, they are concrete proof that your efforts are not in vain. Value these victories and let them propel you to push further.

And when the road seems tough, remember, you're not in this alone. Reach out to loved ones or even online communities for support and encouragement. You'll be amazed at the number of people navigating similar paths, all eager to share their experiences and cheer you on.

Finally, I'd like to leave you with this thought: It's never too late to start living your best life. While age brings challenges, it also imparts wisdom, experience, and a deeper appreciation of what truly matters. By taking responsibility for your health, you're not only investing in your own future, but you're also shaping a legacy of well-being for future generations.

Now, step with courage and a heart full of hope. The path to a healthier, happier you are laid out before you. Embrace it, enjoy every moment, and most importantly, take pride in every step you take.

Jackson McNeil
2023

AUTHOR BIO

Jackson McNeil, author, and health expert, channels his diverse experiences from global adventures to enrich his books. Born into a farmer's life in Eastern Oregon, his journey took him from being a star athlete to an accomplished Chemistry and Physics teacher. His educational pursuits didn't stop there. From Eastern Europe to Russia, SE Asia, and the Republic of the Congo, Jackson absorbed a wealth of knowledge that he skillfully intertwines in his works.

A visionary in combating global health issues, Jackson served as the Deputy Director of an anti-AIDS program, lectured on medical businesses patient – employee relations wielding influence in regions burdened with health challenges. His leadership skills transitioned seamlessly into productive careers in real estate, insurance, and sales and marketing. His seminars, brimming with actionable insights, were highly sought-after events in the health industry.

Now residing in the Southwest with his wife and their

beloved chocolate lab, Jackson enjoys reading, travel, and golf-ing, though he playfully self-identifies as "disappointingly aver-age." His newest release, *"Men Over 50 Get Healthy, Steadfast Strategies to Longevity and Aging Well,"* embodies his personal and professional journeys, offering readers a nuanced approach to wellness, inspired by his life's vast panorama.

REFERENCES

American Cancer Society. (n.d.). American Cancer Society Recommendations for Prostate Cancer Early Detection. Retrieved from https://www.cancer.org/cancer/types/prostate-cancer/detection-diagnosis-staging/acs-recommendations.html

American Heart Association. (n.d.). American Heart Association Recommendations for Physical Activity in Adults and Kids. Retrieved from https://www.heart.org/en/healthy-living/fitness/fitness-basics/aha-recs-for-physical-activity-in-adults

American Heart Association. (n.d.). Staying motivated for fitness. Retrieved from https://www.heart.org/en/healthy-living/fitness/staying-motivated-for-fitness

American Heart Association. (2021). Understand Your Risks to Prevent a Heart Attack. Retrieved from https://www.heart.org/en/health-topics/heart-attack/understand-your-risks-to-prevent-a-heart-attack

American Heart Association. (n.d.). Understanding Blood Pressure Readings. Retrieved from https://www.heart.org/en/health-topics/high-blood-pressure/understanding-blood-pressure-readings

American Psychological Association. (2020). Working out boosts brain health. Retrieved from https://www.apa.org/topics/exercise-fitness/stress

Anderson, E., & Shivakumar, G. (2013). Effects of Exercise and Physical Activity on Anxiety. Frontiers in Psychiatry, 4, 27. https://doi.org/10.3389/fpsyt.2013.00027

ASQ. (n.d.). What is Root Cause Analysis (RCA)? Retrieved from https://asq.org/quality-resources/root-cause-analysis

Avena, N. (n.d.). Not all sleep is restorative — what to know about improving your rest. Healthline. Retrieved from https://www.healthline.com/health/sleep/restorative-sleep

Ayalon, L. (2018). There is nothing new under the sun: Ageism and intergenerational tension in the age of the Anthropocene. European Journal of Ageing, 15(4), 361-368. https://link.springer.com/article/10.1134/S2079057021020089

Barrett, A. E., & Toothman, E. L. (2016). Explaining age differences in women's emotional well-being: The role of subjective experiences of aging. Journal of Women & Aging, 28(4), 285-296. https://journals.sagepub.com/doi/abs/10.2190/1U69-9AU2-V6LH-9Y1L?journalCode=ahdb

Better Health Channel. (n.d.). Physical activity - overcoming excuses. Retrieved from https://www.betterhealth.vic.gov.au/health/healthyliving/Physical-activity-whats-your-excuse

Biddle, S. J., & Asare, M. (2011). Physical activity and mental health in children and adolescents: a review of reviews. British Journal of Sports Medicine, 45(11), 886–895. https://doi.org/10.1136/bjsports-2011-090185

BMC Geriatrics. (2021). Study on aging fears and ways to overcome them. Retrieved from https://www.bmcgeriatrics.com/study-aging-fears

Bokhari, D. (n.d.). 8 Things That Cause Your Lack of Motivation (And How to Fix Them). Retrieved from https://www.deanbokhari.com/lack-of-motivation/

Bromberg-Martin, E. S., Matsumoto, M., & Hikosaka, O. (2010). Dopamine in motivational control: Rewarding, aversive, and alerting. Neuron, 68(5), 815-834. https://doi.org/10.1016/j.neuron.2010.11.022

https://www.youtube.com/watch?v=2XecbuI-9QE

Buijze, G. A., Sierevelt, I. N., van der Heijden, B. C. J. M., Dijkgraaf, M. G., & Frings-Dresen, M. H. W. (2016). The Effect of Cold Showering on Health and Work: A Randomized Controlled Trial. PLoS ONE, 11(9), e0161749. https://doi.org/10.1371/journal.pone.0161749

CDC. (n.d.). About Heart Disease. Retrieved from https://www.cdc.gov/heartdisease/about.htm

CDC. (2021). Estimates of antibiotic-resistant infections and deaths in the United States. Retrieved from https://www.cdc.gov/antibiotic-use/community/for-patients/common-illnesses/antibiotic-resistance.html

CDC. (n.d.). High Blood Pressure Symptoms and Causes. Retrieved from https://www.cdc.gov/bloodpressure/about.htm

CDC. (n.d.). LDL and HDL Cholesterol and Triglycerides. Retrieved from https://www.cdc.gov/cholesterol/ldl_hdl.htm

CDC. (2021). Physical Activity Guidelines for Americans. Retrieved from https://www.cdc.gov/

Centers for Disease Control and Prevention. (n.d.). How much physical activity do older adults need? Retrieved from https://www.cdc.gov/physicalactivity/basics/older_adults/index.htm

Centers for Disease Control and Prevention. (2018). Prevalence of chronic pain and high-impact chronic pain among adults — United States, 2016. Retrieved from https://www.cdc.gov/mmwr/volumes/67/wr/mm6736a2.htm

Cherry, K., & Blackmer, N. (n.d.). 4 stages of sleep: NREM, REM, and the sleep cycle. Verywell Health. Retrieved from https://www.verywellhealth.com/the-four-stages-of-sleep-2795920

Cleveland Clinic. (n.d.). Dopamine: What It Is, Function & Symptoms. Retrieved from https://my.clevelandclinic.org/health/articles/22581-dopamine

Cleveland Clinic. (2021). Why and how you should exercise with arthritis. Retrieved from https://health.clevelandclinic.org/6-ways-to-exercise-with-arthritis/

Coleman, L. M., & Kim, Y. (2016). Gender differences in the perceived threat of aging among midlife women. Journal of Women & Aging, 28(1), 32-43. https://journals.sagepub.com/doi/abs/10.2190/1U69-9AU2-V6LH-9Y1L?journalCode=ahdb

Dana Foundation. (n.d.). How Does Exercise Affect the Brain? Retrieved from https://www.dana.org/article/how-does-exercise-affect-the-brain/

Difference Between: Healthy Aging vs Unhealthy Aging: https://www.differencebetween.net/miscellaneous/difference-between-healthy-aging-and-unhealthy-aging/

Dweck, C. (2016). What Having a "Growth Mindset" Actually Means. Harvard Business Review. Retrieved from https://hbr.org/2016/01/what-having-a-growth-mindset-actually-means

Fox, K. R., Stathi, A., McKenna, J., & Davis, M. G. (2007). Physical activity and mental well-being in older people participating in the Better Ageing Project. European Journal of Applied Physiology, 100(5), 591-602.

Friedman, D. B., & Laditka, S. B. (2011). Advertising and health communication: A content analysis of healthy aging messages in television commercials. Health Communication, 26(6), 546-553. https://pubmed.ncbi.nlm.nih.gov/33272447/

Geneen, L. J., Moore, R. A., Clarke, C., Martin, D., Colvin, L. A., & Smith, B. H. (2017). Physical activity and exercise for chronic pain in adults: an overview of Cochrane Reviews. Cochrane Database of Systematic Reviews, 2017(4), CD011279. https://doi.org/10.1002/14651858.CD011279.pub3

Greater Good Science Center at UC Berkeley. (n.d.). Five Surprising Ways Exercise Changes Your Brain. Retrieved from https://greatergood.berkeley.edu/article/item/five_surprising_ways_exercise_changes_your_brain

Harvard Business Review. (2016). Your Desire to Get Things Done Can Undermine Your Effectiveness. Retrieved from https://hbr.org/2016/03/your-desire-to-get-things-done-can-undermine-your-effectiveness

Harvard Health Publishing. (2021). Does exercise really boost energy levels? Retrieved from https://www.health.harvard.edu/exercise-and-fitness/does-exercise-really-boost-energy-levels

Harvard Medical School. (2019). Foods that fight inflammation. Retrieved from https://www.health.harvard.edu/staying-healthy/foods-that-fight-inflammation

Harvard Health Publishing. (2021). How much exercise do you need? Retrieved from https://www.health.harvard.edu/exercise-and-fitness/how-much-exercise-do-you-need

Harvard Health Publishing. (2018). Overcome exercise excuses. Retrieved from https://www.health.harvard.edu/blog/overcome-exercise-excuses-2018042113685

Harvard Health Publishing. (2020). Understanding the stress response - Harvard Health. Retrieved from https://www.health.harvard.edu/staying-healthy/understanding-the-stress-response

Harvard Health Publishing. (2019, November 28). Will a purpose-driven life help you live longer? Retrieved from https://www.health.harvard.edu/blog/will-a-purpose-driven-life-help-you-live-longer-2019112818378

Healthfully. (n.d.). What Triggers Dopamine? Retrieved from https://healthfully.com/what-triggers-dopamine-5751760.html

Healthline. (n.d.). HDL vs. LDL Cholesterol: What's the Difference? Retrieved from https://www.healthline.com/health/hdl-vs-ldl-cholesterol

Innerbody Research. (n.d.). Mental health benefits of exercise. Retrieved from https://www.innerbody.com/mental-health-benefits-of-exercise

International Journal of Aging and Human Development. (2022). [Gender differences in anxiety about aging]. Retrieved from https://www.internationaljournalofagingandhumandevelopment.com/anxiety-aging-gender-differences

Into Action Recovery Centers. (n.d.). Effects of Dopamine: How Dopamine Drives Human Behavior. Retrieved from https://www.intoactionrecovery.com/how-dopamine-drives-our-behavior/

Institute of Medicine (US) Committee on Sleep Medicine and Research. (2006). Sleep Disorders and Sleep Deprivation: An Unmet Public Health Problem. National Academies Press (US). Retrieved from https://www.ncbi.nlm.nih.gov/

Jones, A. (2020). The double standard of aging theory. Journal of Women & Aging, 35(2), 145-163.

JNCI: Journal of the National Cancer Institute. (2003). Tomatoes or Lycopene Versus Prostate Cancer: Is Evolution Anti-Reductionist? Retrieved from https://academic.oup.com/jnci/article/95/21/1563/2520528

Kotwal, A., & Fan, J. (2020). Double Standard of Aging Theory: A Critical Perspective. Journal of gerontological nursing, 46(1), 25-31. https://pubmed.ncbi.nlm.nih.gov/33272447/

Kox, M., van Eijk, L. T., Zwaag, J., van den Wildenberg, J., Sweep, F. C. G. J., van der Hoeven, J. G., & Pickkers, P. (2014). Voluntary activation of the sympathetic nervous system and attenuation of the innate immune response in humans. Proceedings of the National Academy of Sciences, 111(20), 7379–7384. https://doi.org/10.1073/pnas.1322174111

Leaders First. (2019). 10 Ways to Improve Productivity with Dopamine. Retrieved from https://leadersfirst.org/10-ways-to-improve-productivity-with-dopamine/

Litvinenko, I. V., & Ivanova, A. E. (2018). Fear of aging and ways to overcome it. Advances in gerontology – Uspekhi gerontologii, 31(5), 657-662. https://www.ncbi.nlm.nih.gov/pmc/articles/PMC6011296/

Manual. (n.d.). Normal Testosterone Levels by Age. Retrieved from https://www.manual.co/health-centre/testosterone/normal-testosterone-levels-by-age

Mayo Clinic. (n.d.). Blood pressure chart: What your reading means. Retrieved from https://www.mayoclinic.org/diseases-conditions/high-blood-pressure/in-depth/blood-pressure/art-20050982

Mayo Clinic. (n.d.). Erectile dysfunction - Symptoms and causes. Retrieved from https://www.mayoclinic.org/diseases-conditions/erectile-dysfunction/symptoms-causes/syc-20355776

Mayo Clinic. (n.d.). Exercising with arthritis: Improve your joint pain and stiffness. Retrieved from https://www.mayoclinic.org/diseases-conditions/arthritis/in-depth/arthritis/art-20047971

Mayo Clinic. (2021). High blood pressure (hypertension). Retrieved from https://www.mayoclinic.org/diseases-conditions/high-blood-pressure/symptoms-causes/syc-20373410

Mayo Clinic. (n.d.). Sleep disorders - Symptoms and causes. Retrieved from https://www.mayoclinic.org/diseases-conditions/sleep-disorders/symptoms-causes/syc-20354018

Mayo Clinic. (2021). Sleep tips: 6 steps to better sleep. Retrieved from https://www.mayoclinic.org/healthy-lifestyle/adult-health/in-depth/sleep/art-20048379

Medical News Today. (2018). 9 best exercises for rheumatoid arthritis pain. Retrieved from https://www.medicalnewstoday.com/articles/322917

Mental Health Daily. (2015). How To Increase Dopamine Levels. Retrieved from https://mentalhealthdaily.com/2015/04/17/how-to-increase-dopamine-levels/

Merck Manual. (2020). Adverse effects of excessive medication use. Retrieved from https://www.merckmanuals.com/home/drugs/adverse-drug-reactions/adverse-effects-of-excessive-medication-use

Merck Manual: Aging and Medications. https://www.merckmanuals.-

com/home/older-people%E2%80%99s-health-issues/aging-and-medica-tions/aging-and-medications

National Cancer Institute. (n.d.). Understanding Prostate Changes: A Health Guide for Men. Retrieved from https://www.cancer.gov/types/prostate/understanding-prostate-changes

National Institute on Aging. (2020). Exercise and Physical Activity. Retrieved from https://www.nia.nih.gov/health/topics/exercise-and-physical-activity

National Institute on Aging. (n.d.). What do we know about healthy aging? https://www.nia.nih.gov/health/what-do-we-know-about-healthy-aging

National Institute on Aging. Exercise and physical activity: Your everyday guide from the National Institute on Aging https://www.nia.nih.gov/health/topics/exercise-and-physical-activity

National Institute on Aging. (n.d.). Participating in activities you enjoy as you age. Retrieved from https://www.nia.nih.gov/health/participating-activities-you-enjoy-you-age

National Institute on Aging. (n.d.). Staying Motivated to Exercise: Tips for Older Adults. Retrieved from https://www.nia.nih.gov/health/staying-motivated-exercise-tips-older-adults

National Institutes of Health. (2020). Chronic Pain: Symptoms, Diagnosis, & Treatment. Retrieved from https://www.nccih.nih.gov/health/chronic-pain-what-you-need-to-know

NHLBI. (n.d.). DASH Eating Plan. Retrieved from https://www.nhlbi.nih.gov/education/dash-eating-plan

NIMH. (2019). Older Adults and Mental Health. Retrieved from https://www.nimh.nih.gov/

Niv, Y., Daw, N. D., & Dayan, P. (2005). How fast to work: Response vigor, motivation, and tonic dopamine. In Advances in Neural Information Processing Systems 18 (NIPS 2005) (pp. 1019-1026). MIT Press.

Ontario CMHA. (n.d.). Connection between mental and physical health. Retrieved from https://ontario.cmha.ca/documents/connection-between-mental-and-physical-health/

Penedo, F. J., & Dahn, J. R. (2005). Exercise and well-being: a review of mental and physical health benefits associated with physical activity. Current Opinion in Psychiatry, 18(2), 189–193. https://doi.org/10.1097/00001504-200503000-00013

Pinto Pereira, S. M., Geoffroy, M. C., & Power, C. (2014). Depressive Symptoms and Physical Activity During 3 Decades in Adult Life: Bidirectional Associations in a Prospective Cohort Study. JAMA Psychiatry, 71(12), 1373–1380. https://doi.org/10.1001/jamapsychiatry.2014.1240

Psychology Today. (n.d.). Growth Mindset. Retrieved from https://www.psychologytoday.com/us/basics/growth-mindset

Rosenblatt, C. (2022, June 20). Are You Setting Yourself Up For Unhealthy Aging? Forbes. https://www.forbes.com/sites/carolynrosenblatt/2022/06/20/are-you-setting-yourself-up-for-unhealthy-aging/?sh=475514e312a2

Jones, A., & Smith, B. (2018). Root Cause Analysis: Uncovering the Underlying Factors of Problems. Journal of Problem Solving, 30(2), 125-140.

Salamone, J. D., & Correa, M. (2012). The mysterious motivational functions of mesolimbic dopamine. Neuron, 76(3), 470-485. https://doi.org/10.1016/j.neuron.2012.10.021

Schultz, W. (2015). Neuronal reward and decision signals: From theories to data. Physiological Reviews, 95(3), 853-951. https://doi.org/10.1152/physrev.00023.2014

Shevchuk, N. A. (2008). Adapted cold shower as a potential treatment for depression. Medical Hypotheses, 70(5), 995–1001. https://doi.org/10.1016/j.mehy.2007.04.052

Sleep Foundation. (n.d.). Sleep disorders – Common types, symptoms, treatments. Retrieved from https://www.sleepfoundation.org/sleep-disorders

Smith, A., Johnson, L., & Davis, R. (2022). The impact of unhappiness on physical and mental health. Journal of Happiness Studies, 19(4), 1345-1362.

Smith, J., Johnson, L. M., & Brown, L. M. (2019). Unhealthy aging: Causes and consequences. Journal of Aging and Health, 31(8), 1469-1487.

The American Institute of Stress. (2021). The Physical Effects of Long-Term Stress. Retrieved from https://www.stress.org/

The Lancet Public Health. (2020). The value of maintaining social connections for mental health in older people. Retrieved from https://www.thelancet.com/journals/lanpub/article/PIIS2468-2667%2819%2930253-1/fulltext

Time. (n.d.). How to Break Bad Habits, According to Science. Retrieved from https://time.com/5373528/break-bad-habit-science/

University of Rochester Medical Center. (2021). Why Exercise and Sleep Are Your Ultimate Defense Against Stress. Retrieved from https://www.urmc.rochester.edu/

UpToDate. (n.d.). Patient education: Arthritis and exercise (Beyond the Basics). Retrieved from https://www.uptodate.com/contents/arthritis-and-exercise-beyond-the-basics

Verywell Mind. (n.d.). Neuroplasticity: How Experience Changes the Brain. Retrieved from https://www.verywellmind.com/what-is-brain-plasticity-2794886

Walker, T. (2023). Boosting physical activity may ease chronic pain. Medical News Today. Retrieved from https://www.medicalnewstoday.com/articles/becoming-more-physically-active-linked-to-higher-pain-tolerance

Wise, R. A. (2013). Dual roles of dopamine in food and drug seeking: the drive-reward paradox. Biological Psychiatry, 73(9), 819-826. https://doi.org/10.1016/j.biopsych.2012.09.001

Working Partners. (n.d.). America's prescription drug abuse epidemic: A quick-fix mentality. https://www.workingpartners.com/americas-prescription-drug-abuse-epidemic-quick-fix-mentality/

Working Partners. (2021). Report on prescription painkiller consumption in the United States. Retrieved from https://www.workingpartners.com/painkiller-consumption-report

World Health Organization. (2020). Physical Activity. Retrieved from https://www.who.int/

Zotova, E. V., & Steblovskaya, A. V. (2021). Fear of aging: Emotional, cognitive, and behavioral aspects. Advances in Gerontology, 11(1), 33-43. https://www.ncbi.nlm.nih.gov/pmc/articles/PMC6011296/

www.ingramcontent.com/pod-product-compliance
Lightning Source LLC
Chambersburg PA
CBHW060452280326
41933CB00014B/2734